WOMB LIFE

WONDERS AND CHALLENGES OF PREGNANCY, THE FOETUS' JOURNEY AND BIRTH

GRAHAM MUSIC

MIND-NURTURING BOOKS

Published in 2024 by Mind-Nurturing Books

90 Huddleston Road, London, N7 0EG

British Library Cataloguing-in-Publication Data

A catalogue record for this book is available from the British Library

ISBN: (pbk) 978-1-7398147-6-2

ISBN: (ebk) 978-1-7398147-7-9

ISBN: (hbk) 978-1-7398147-8-6

This is, without doubt, the most important book on pregnancy and 'womb life' I've ever read. It's rich in scientific detail, yet accessible and interesting. I followed the foetuses' journey gripped. Graham Music is a colossus in the world of child psychotherapy. I only wish he had written this book twenty years ago when I was pregnant! **Annalisa Barbieri, Guardian columnist and podcaster**

Graham Music has crafted an immensely readable book, richly infused with the voices and experiences of parents and professionals yet intertwined with accessible explanations of contemporary scientific research. This book will deepen your knowledge about the emotional and physical transitions to babyhood and parenthood and will be of interest to anyone connected to the experiences of pregnancy, birth and bonding". **Dr Karen Bateson, Joint CEO, Oxford Parent-Infant Project**

Very accessible, amazingly comprehensive, fascinating, and a delight to read. This book opens a clear and comprehensive window into the hidden world of the womb. Music wonderfully weaves together, in the most accessible way, the psychoanalytic, neurological, cultural, psychological, recent research findings, and most importantly the deeply personal accounts of mothers-to-be. He illuminates this world with his typical breath of understanding, humour, empathy, and lovely personal touches. It is a "must have" for not only parents-to-be but also any professionals dealing with the mental health of a child, adolescent, or adult. This addition to the literature greatly deepens our understanding of this "beyond words" world. **Peter Blake, Director and Founder of the Institute of Child and Adolescent Psychoanalytic Psychotherapy, Sydney, and author of Child and Adolescent Psychotherapy (3rd ed 2021)**

We have learnt so much in recent decades about Child and Infant Mental Health, and now Graham Music has gone deeper still with his interest in pregnancy and the foetus. With this book, many mothers will be helped to deal with the complexities of pregnancy, and many babies should be grateful that they were thought about well before they were born. **Dilys Daws, Consultant Psychotherapist, Tavistock Clinic, Founder of the Association of Infant Mental Health, UK and author of Parent-Infant Psychotherapy for Sleep problems (2020) and Finding Your Way with your Baby (2021)**

TABLE OF CONTENTS

DEDICATION

To my mother, who carried me inside her when she was not much more than a child herself, and who brought me into the world, in pain, from her own flesh, and with love. Thank you.

ACKNOWLEDGEMENTS

With deep appreciation to the many who have helped me try to make sense of pregnancy and life in the womb, none of whom are responsible in any way for anything in the text! These include:

Nikita Akilapa, Annalisa Barbieri, Sue Beecraft, Debbie Brace, Annabelle Chown, Laura Condell, Dagmar Field, Tafi Gashi, Rob Glanz, Patrick Heaney, Jessica James, Shivani Lamba, Rose Beecraft Music, Rajinder Keohane, Kate Lucre, Amanda Bueno de Mesquita, Jess Murray, India Rakusen, Maria Rathay, Jane O'Rourke, Sally O'Rourke, Karina Sarmiento, Mia Von Scha, Kesella Scott-Somme, Jo Violet, Bianca Zorz.

Thanks too to Klara and Eric King for exceptional copy-editing once again, to Xee Shan for both cover design and formatting and to Dania Awan for proof-reading and indexing.

ABOUT THE AUTHOR

Graham Music (PHD) is an author, psychotherapist, keynote speaker, trainer, and supervisor. In his younger days, his work included antique dealing, supporting the homeless, and even house renovation. He was until recently Consultant Child and Adolescent Psychotherapist at the Tavistock Centre in London, where he worked for over 25 years, and he has had an adult psychotherapy practice for over 35 years. Formerly Associate Clinical Director of the Tavistock Clinic's Child and Family Department, his passion and clinical experience has been in working with trauma, especially at the Tavistock's Fostering and Adoption and Kinship Care team and at various child mental health teams and at the Portman Clinic.

He has developed and managed a range of services working with the aftermath of child maltreatment and neglect and has prioritized community-based services for people who are often marginalized from mainstream clinic work, including developing services in over forty schools.

He supervises and teaches on a range of trainings in the UK, delivers many keynote talks at conferences, and often teaches internationally – for example, in Sicily, Istanbul, Iceland, Hong Kong, Finland, Canada, South Africa, and Australia.

He has a particular interest in linking cutting-edge developmental findings with therapeutic practice. His publications include *Nurturing Natures* (2024, 2016, 2010), *Affect and Emotion* (2023, 2001), *Respark: Igniting Hope and Joy after Trauma and Depression* (2022), *Nurturing Children: From*

Trauma to Hope (2019), *The Good Life* (2014), and *From Trauma to Harming Others* (co-edited with Ariel Nathanson and Janine Sternberg, 2021).

The Chief Executive of the Anna Freud Centre, Professor Peter Fonagy OBE, wrote about the book *Nurturing Children* that Graham Music is 'certainly one of the best, and probably the most deep-thinking, child psychotherapists in the world … this book is a must.'

And attachment expert Professor Jeremy Holmes stated that 'Music is the David Attenborough of child development research.'

———— ··●·· ————

Find out more about his work from his website *https://nurturingnatures.co.uk/* or use this QR to access.

Do sign up for Graham Music's newsletter, which includes many goodies such as blogs, publications, and forthcoming courses and events *https://nurturingnatures.co.uk/sign-up/* or using this QR code.

PREFACE

It is with great excitement that we, the editorial board of Mind-Nurturing Books, introduce this beautifully written book on prenatal life and pregnancy. This is the first in a series of guides by Dr Graham Music, each focusing on a key aspect of child development. This volume looks at the very beginnings of life, at pregnancy, and the foetus' journey. We hear about some mind-blowing science, cross-cultural understandings, and about what most increases the chances of a smooth pregnancy and birth. The book and themes are brought to life by the voices of women who tell their stories with honesty and generosity.

At a time when mental health issues are skyrocketing, understanding how children grow, learn, and thrive has never been more important, and this includes understanding the very start of life. The fields of developmental science have uncovered extraordinary new insights that can help us support our children's emotional, psychological, and educational needs. All too often, this vital knowledge remains locked away in academic texts where it is hard to find for those who would most benefit from it. Graham Music has had a lifelong passion to demystify such scientific research and make it accessible through his writing, speaking, and courses. Complex concepts, from the building blocks of the brain to the formation of emotional bonds, to the effects of stress and trauma, to the importance of cross-cultural understanding, are all made readily accessible here and in his other writing.

We read insightful and moving clinical and personal stories, alongside evidence-based approaches for helping children flourish. Continuing the themes of his best-selling book, Nurturing Natures, Music examines the interplay between innate inherited capacities and environmental influences. Parents, educators, and mental health professionals will find a treasure trove of fascinating information to apply in their interactions with parents and children.

We have called the books in this series 'guides', not because they are full of advice or 'how to do things' information; rather, we see them as being more like maps that contain the information needed for readers, whether professionals, parents, or interested lay people, to navigate and make the best sense they can of the terrain, and so help them find the most appropriate way to go on their own journey.

This volume, like all of Graham Music's work, is written in a readable and human style, but without shirking difficult issues or the complexity of the debates. You will receive reliable information based on the latest science and research, alongside time-honoured knowledge, longstanding therapeutic and personal experience, and an awareness of contemporary issues, including race, gender, and neurodiversity, as well as the wisdom of other cultures and societies. This book starts right at the beginning of life, and other books will take this forward with topics such as the capacities of the new baby, the primary-aged child, stress and becoming resilient, the role of play, the importance of cultural differences, understanding the brain and nervous system, trauma and neglect, as well as fathers and childcare.

Mind-Nurturing books aim to help anyone involved in the care of tomorrow's citizens to optimise their potential.

Science, alongside clinical wisdom and cultural understanding can unlock new possibilities for those caring for our next generation. As Graham Music says, 'We need to know what the science really shows, and also gather the insights of clinicians and parents and the wisdom of other cultures, but I also hope readers will use these books as a springboard to trust their own instincts and hearts and to follow their inner guides.'

We hope you enjoy the journey!

Editorial team, Mind-Nurturing Books, March 2024

Jane O'Rourke, child, adolescent, and family psychotherapist and Founder of MINDinMIND.

Shivani Lamba, neuroscience expert, international leader in using tech to enhance children's wellbeing, and founder of Brightlobe.

A NOTE ON LANGUAGE, QUOTES, AND REFERENCING

Language that until recently was taken for granted is nowadays being contested. In the world of parenting and childcare, perhaps the strongest debates are around gender identity and biological sex. I have questioned how ok it is these days to even use the word 'mother' as opposed to 'birthgiver' or 'pregnant person', and, of course, what pronouns to use. The last thing I want to do is to offend anyone, but it is also impossible to please everyone. True, many trans men were born with two X chromosomes and still have a womb and can and do get pregnant, and I agree that all parents deserve to have their identity acknowledged and respected. Yet the vast majority of people who give birth do identify as female and cherish thinking of themselves as mothers. For so many, being a mother is an important part of their identity, something they feel proud of and that they want to be acknowledged. Hence, in the spirit of compromise, I have used mainly the terms 'mother' and 'woman', but sometimes more gender-neutral terms, such as birthgiver, or birthing or pregnant person. I really hope that readers will take this in the spirit intended.

You will see that the themes in each chapter are brought to life with quotations from women I have interviewed. I have sometimes changed the names, but the content has been either quoted verbatim or slightly adjusted to ensure confidentiality. I am incredibly grateful to have these voices bringing the science alive.

Finally, I have tried to make this book as readable as I could, but I also want to give people the chance to look up the evidence on which I have based it, which is mostly from peer-reviewed academic papers or books by distinguished researchers and clinicians. I have placed a number after each source with a matching reference at the end of the book. So, only for those so inclined, happy researching!

CHAPTER 1

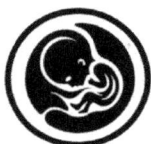

INTRODUCTION

I assume you are reading this guide because someone – perhaps you, or a loved one, or a client or someone you are responsible for – is pregnant or hoping to have a baby. There is so much to learn and make sense of, and it is easy to lose one's bearings.

One reason for writing this book is that our knowledge-base has moved forward so much in recent decades. There is also much wisdom to reclaim from other cultures, much of which is in danger of being forgotten. Yet we are faced with an overabundance of conflicting opinions, plus much misinformation that can evoke fear, shame, and anxiety. In the contemporary world, there is terrible pressure on parents: it is all too easy to feel guilty, and it is hard to know where to turn or what to trust.

This guide sets out to redress this. I use clinical and personal stories of women and professionals, alongside the latest science as well as cross-cultural understanding, all with the aim of helping women and babies have the best experience possible, and to try to set the healthiest foundations for later life.

It might seem strange that I, a man, am writing about pregnancy and birth. I certainly had some misgivings about doing so. After all, I can never give birth, and my pain thresholds match the classic caricature of men who shriek at a splinter or moan at man-flu. This book, though, is the first of a series of short guides about children's development, and it seemed odd not to start at the very beginning of life. I hope it is the voices of women and professionals in the field that clearly shine through, alongside amazing and important facts about the foetus and pregnancy.

I do have a personal investment in this subject. I am a father, have witnessed birth, and have worked with many pregnant women, as well as with too many children and adults whose lives in the womb had adversely affected them. Also, my own early life origins – indeed, my own life before birth – have given rise to issues that affect me to this day.

I often think back to the cultural consensus in the United Kingdom way back at the time of my own birth, and the effects of this on newborns. My own mother had no preparation at all for my birth and, indeed, had not even been told that the process was going to be painful! She went through labour with no support, with no one with her whom she knew; my father was absent at a cricket match, and, anyway, partners were rarely present at births in those days. It was a long, difficult labour, my mother was unconscious when I was born, and doctors used a Ventouse (a kind of vacuum suction cap) to pull me out; indeed, my adult bald head still bears the scars! My mother was sedated, while I was subjected to various medical procedures and then placed in a cot in a room with other cots, each containing another distressed baby who was brought out every few hours for food or occasional holding. The process was based absolutely on a medical model in which white coats, scrupulous hygiene, and safety were a far higher priority than emotional support or understanding.

In that bygone era, when I started out as a foetus and infant, and indeed when I started practising as a therapist, about 35 years ago, there was barely any understanding that life before birth was even important! How little we knew, and what a loss that is for so many people we worked with at that time!

New babies, and indeed unborn babies, are society's most precious resources. We need to learn how to give our children the best chance to flourish. Thankfully in the decades since my 1950s birth we have learnt so much that is vital, and in this short guide I highlight, with the help of colleagues and experts, as well as stories from generous women 'experts by experience', what I believe is most helpful to think about.

Every single pregnancy will be experienced differently by both foetus and mother. Rarely do events unfold as swimmingly as pregnancy books, healthcare professionals, or social media influencers suggest. How things go will depend on so many different factors, such as how much support is around, the parents' states of mind, the quality of their relationships, their culture, their personal histories, as well as plain luck of the draw, including biology and genes. Here are two very different examples.

Jinji told me:

> *It had taken me years to know I even wanted a baby, and I did not think I was mother material; my own childhood had been very complicated. When we first decided to give it a go, I*

was not holding my breath. But I know, just know, I got pregnant the very first time we tried. I sat in my work toilet with the test result in my hand, confirming what my whole being already knew: 'This changes everything'. From those first moments I was in a new sort of love, transported, dreamy, more protective than I had ever felt, excited, nervous, but gloriously happy. It probably sounds mad, but we talked, I stroked him (I just knew it was a him), and I felt a new kind of euphoric bliss, as if, despite my successful career and material success, my whole life had been awaiting these moments and this unfolding future. As the months went by, I felt I knew him better than I had known anyone, and also that he knew me. It sounds strange, I know, but I was transformed and had become what I thought I would never be: an example of archetypal all-consuming mother love!

Of course, it is not always so simple, as in the case of Annabel Chown, a writer and gifted yoga teacher whose classes I have attended for years:

It took me five years from deciding I wanted to have a baby to becoming pregnant. My husband and I eventually conceived via our third and what we agreed would be a final round of IVF. The clinic where we'd had that round of IVF told me to take a pregnancy test 11 days after my embryo transfer. I woke around 3 am on the day, and knowing it was the day I needed to test, I knew there was no way I'd be able to go back to sleep and wait until morning properly came around. I didn't wake my husband – he hates being woken up, and I also knew that, at the time, he was less invested in being a parent than I was, so wouldn't mind if I'd tested without him by my side. I knew the test could take up to 3 minutes to show a result, so I went into the kitchen to get a glass of water. When I came back, I was, to be honest, expecting to see a negative test result, so was totally shocked to see two clear blue lines.

Adrenaline raced through me, a feeling that continued throughout that day – which happened to be a bright and beautiful mid-April day in London. I called the clinic to tell them the result, and they told me I needed to go and get a blood test done, to check my hormones and see how viable the pregnancy looked. I walked through the local park to get the test done. Everything was in bloom, and I felt full of joy and excitement. Also, of course, there was some fear. What if the pregnancy proved not to be viable? The blood test came back showing great hormones, so I relaxed a little.

A week later, I was alone at home on a Sunday morning (my husband was away for the weekend) when I started bleeding. How could I have dared think this would work, I thought to myself. That's it. The end of this long-awaited dream.

'You need a scan', the clinic told me, 'to check whether the pregnancy is still viable. We simply can't know without one.' Except I'd have to wait until the end of the week for a scan, as it was too early to have one yet. Those were the longest five days. I walked through the same park, still in its spring glory, and tried not to think about the worst possibility. I tried to just stay present to what was right in front of me. Which was hard.

On the day of the scan, I was shaking. I'd also prepared for the worst. The thump-thump of the heartbeat shocked me. Made me cry.

After that, I was, for the first few weeks, wary. Would this happen again? Would it be over next time? And when morning sickness didn't come, I panicked. I had heard it was a 'good sign' of a strong pregnancy. So perhaps I wasn't even pregnant *anymore? I insisted on another scan. The baby was still there, heart still beating away.*

The nausea never came, and gradually the fear eased, not least from having had 12- and then 20-week scans where I was told everything was looking good. And much as nausea may have given me some psychological reassurance, what a gift it was to have an easeful pregnancy, where I felt really well in my body. It helped make the pregnancy, after those first anxious weeks, a really joyful experience for me, a time I look back on as a very happy one.'

We will hear many more stories from Annabelle and other women as we go along.

What's in the book?

In chapter 2, I go over some of the most fascinating facts about what exactly happens from conception through to the time of birth, including some of the surprising things a foetus can do and experience. We see what an extraordinary being the foetus is, what astonishing capacities it has to get what it needs and the myriad ways in which it interacts with its host, and we learn about some of the things it can do from really early on in its existence. Central to this guide is a simple idea: that the not-yet-born baby is both an autonomous being and also totally dependent; it is making sense of its world, adapting to it, even making decisions, but always picking up messages from its milieu, mainly the mother, and responding to those.

In chapter 3 I continue this theme through the lens of what we learn from ultrasound scans (a lot in fact), before thinking briefly in chapter 4 about the phenomenal growth of millions of brain cells and the burgeoning mental capacities that appear well before birth.

Next, in chapter 5, 'Wow or Woo?', we open up the world of prenatal bonding, which can sometimes be seen as slightly left-field. I hope to convince you of just how important such bonding can be for setting up the foundations for good, attuned, and loving later experiences. We dive into sometimes mind-blowing examples of connections between mothers and their unborn babies. Can the mother communicate with the foetus, and does the foetus respond to this, and how important is such bonding for later communication? The themes in this chapter echo those in the whole book: that it is the experience of good emotional connection, of feeling safe in the presence of another person or, indeed, of several people, or, better, a community, of feeling trust and ease, that leads to emotional and physical health. All this most certainly can start in utero.

Next, in chapter 6, I take up the important issue of culture and indigenous knowledge, unpacking a theme that infuses the book: that we can and should learn so much from other cultures. I ask whether we have thrown away important ancient wisdom in embracing the very real gains of Western science. After all, humans have always given birth and we have learnt a thing or two over the millennia, and there might be costs to forgetting such ancient knowledge.

We will see how, in many cultures, women preparing for childbirth benefited from advice and stories handed down by elder women. It is true that infant mortality has lessened considerably in modern times, but in the transition from such oral traditions to a medical hospital-based model, it is possible that a lot has been lost as well as gained.[1] Historically, pregnancy and birth were part of socio-spiritual traditions, wrapped in ritual and tradition. Of course, we should beware of romanticising traditional ways, which certainly came with risks. A technological birth like mine would not have been possible in any culture in human history before the last century, and there is a good chance that before such modern medicine, both my mother and I might not have survived. But we can also become aware of what has been lost – not least the sense of belonging, community, intergenerational cultural and spiritual transmission, and the very real gains of these for the nervous systems of both foetus and mother.

Then, in chapter 7, I talk about what we don't hear about on Instagram or TV parenting programs: that there can be complex and mixed feelings about having a baby and, most importantly, that it is not all about love and bliss. Indeed, ambivalence and negative or difficult feelings are normal and absolutely expectable. I try to look square in the face at what most of us don't like to think about, that being a mother and baby is never just about love, and, yes, conflict and strife are inevitably part of the picture, even at a cellular level. The foetus and the pregnant mother are sharing, and sometimes fighting for, space and resources, and they need to try to find a balance, or homeostasis. The foetus is not just passively bathing in a blissful bath of amniotic fluid. It is active, interactive, and has its own agenda. In fact, it pressures the mother to respond to its needs, and it also very much adapts to and learns from the unique intrauterine environment it finds itself in. This is very much co-regulation, always two-way, each partner profoundly affecting the other.

I then, in chapter 8, look at how parents' psychological histories, and indeed what happened in previous generations, can impact on the developing baby; unfair as it can seem, an unborn baby can pay a price for what their grandparents had experienced. Every foetus and birthgiver – indeed, every one of us – is a product of our cultural heritage, our socioeconomic circumstances, our intergenerational history, our genetic and epigenetic history, and our current influences. Very much in this mix are the influences of life even before conception and before birth, affecting how our very genes get turned on and off.[2] In chapter 8 we learn more about what can seem unfair: that the more adverse childhood experiences, or ACEs, we have, the more the risk to our own and our children's long-term health outcomes.[3] Such adverse experiences are not in the control of parents and might include poverty, inequality, racism, as well as family trauma;[4] these all are likely to have an effect.

In the following chapter, chapter 9, I try to tackle issues that too often concern mothers: the impact of factors like stress, as well as what we take into our bodies, such as nutrients and more worrying substances. I hope to avoid guilt but to also be alert to the foetus's sensitivity and needs. We see how the foetus is swimming in a sea of information about its environment, constantly receiving biochemical and other feedback, and is continually adapting and responding to this. Humans, including foetuses, are always learning, and, as researcher, David Chamberlain said, 'the womb is the first school of life, and we have all attended it'.[5]

This is important as we move into the final two chapters to discuss (deep breath) the big moments of birth, preparation, support, and both what helps this to go smoothly as well as what can go wrong. These chapters probably have more stories from women than the others – after all, we know how storytelling is so important, especially for making sense of birthing experiences, and it is how humans both process experience and learn. An important theme centres around what knowledge and what authority we can trust, and how we can get the best balance between a woman trusting her own body, her intuition and sense of what her baby needs, alongside medical expertise, expectations, and procedures.

Here, as throughout the book, I highlight the absolutely crucial importance of support from others, whether partners, friends, or experienced women such as doulas who really understand the process of birth and who know what can help or hinder a good experience for both mother and baby. Good social connection and feeling safe are always really important – in fact, essential – for human psychological health, perhaps never more so than for a pregnant woman or new mother. Stress and fear, the opposite of feeling safe, can lead to a drawing inward, away from emotional trust and openness, just when we need them most.[6] This book aims to maximise the potential for the opposite: for Positive Childhood Experiences (PCEs), and a sense of safeness and ease, which can begin well before birth.

These chapters just about wind up the book, although at the end I briefly introduce the next volume in the series, which, not surprisingly, is about the first year of life and the extraordinary capacities of the newborn. After all, this is just the beginning.

What I take for granted throughout the book is that, well before birth, we see a being, an organism, that is learning, predicting, and responding, and also clearly has its own agenda. The expectation that we hope is being built in the very cells, psyche, and biology of the foetus is a deep belief that the world they come out into will be one of love, ease, safeness, and pleasure. This guide aims to describe just how we can start to form such good foundations and build hopeful expectations from very early on, well before we are born.

CHAPTER 2

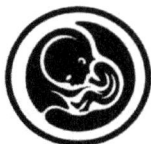

HOW A LIFE STARTS, AND SOME OF WHAT THE FOETUS CAN DO

A new life can begin in so many ways. Take my social work colleague, Claudia:

I had no intention of getting pregnant, had been told over the years by doctors I couldn't, and I was happily determined to focus on my career, helping other people's children at work, on being an aunt and godmother, and to resolutely enjoy a life of adventure. I barely noticed when I missed my first period, and a few weeks later, feeling somewhat nauseous, I was taken aback when my oldest friend asked if I might be pregnant. To say I was shocked to find out would be an understatement! In truth, initially, the news was somewhat unwelcome and threw my life upside down. It took several months to make peace with the idea and begin to accept, and then plan, and only then to start to get really excited. A few months later nothing would have convinced me not to have this precious being, but it could so easily not have been.

Quite different was the story of my colleague from Germany, Maria, who so desperately wanted a baby:

We had been trying for almost five years, and I had already started letting go of hope, with lots of tears and grief, and then I fell pregnant on holiday. I asked my husband to ritually invite the unborn baby into our lives on one of our hikes together. It felt right, and I was sure that the soul was already there.

Before that, I had visited my aunt in the Black Forest. She supported me by doing daily yoga, and she gave me a book about ancient herbs that help conception, and we collected the herbs in the mountains together.

Afterwards, I visited a very good friend, who cried with me about not being able to get pregnant.

This support from other women helped, as did Covid lockdowns, as they slowed me down and reduced my travelling for work. I also did fertility yoga, journaled, and meditated a lot. I had acupuncture, as there wasn't any medical indication that either my husband or I shouldn't get pregnant. I also stopped high-intensity sports and stuck with walks and yoga. I think it was this potpourri of different measures that helped me to get pregnant.

One thing about being pregnant that is absolutely different is that women are no longer in control of their own bodies. They have an experience of something that is often called co-embodiment[7]: the sharing of one's body and bodily functions with another, something we might only otherwise see in, for example, Siamese twins.

If the foetus needs nutrients, then it will do its best to ensure the mother responds to those needs! If a mother is blissed out, the foetus will be swimming in very different chemicals than if the mother is very stressed, and in either case the foetus will be learning from such experiences and developing its own particular expectations. Any foetus, by the time it becomes a newborn baby, has already made specific predictions of what its world is likely to be like, what sounds to expect, what tastes, as well as whether to expect ease and love or, if unlucky, a scarier world. After all, mother and foetus have spent about nine months in extremely close proximity, sharing so many chemicals, fluids, hormones, and more. In effect, mother and foetus are not two beings; they are intersecting and linked, and they mutually interact and, indeed, affect each other at a cellular level.

As my psychiatrist colleague Emily told me:

> *Such a strange sensation to now be two. You think you are stepping into the private spaces of your life, only to realise you are never alone. There is always a something, a someone, an entity, a being. What to make of them? How to converse, to lull, to not feel too shy, to enjoy sharing your space?*

Emily had said:

> *I knew I was pregnant, pretty much at conception. I could feel everything, even an entry of an alien essence that second time … (strange, but true). Then a gradual 'digging-in' sensation over a few days, a little painful even. I didn't really need confirmation, but nonetheless when the little device confirmed the result, an excitement, a giddiness, and a fear gripped – a bit like launching oneself off the top of a rickety helter-skelter.*

> *Then there were the weird sensations of feeling nauseated at times, quite a lot, a metallic taste; a surprising dislike of*

> alcohol, and a general background buzz of something, as if there was a concert of bees working their way into my very cellular structure.

Not everyone's experience is the same, by any means. Here is what Sally experienced, a full 30 years before she became a psychotherapist:

> I was more than four months along when I was shocked to find out I was pregnant. I was just 20. I remember asking my friend if she had had a period and her telling me that was the fourth time I had asked her! I realise in retrospect that the not knowing about the pregnancy was me disassociating and not being able to face reality. I was in a grim situation. I had secretly married a man when I was 18, and my life had no structure and no prospects. I was deeply unhappy and could not bear facing the realisation and consequences of a pregnancy, which I believe would have felt overwhelming. It has taken me until now to realise that abusive experiences in my own childhood had led me to cut off awareness of my bodily feelings and states, something that I am only now recovering from.

Yet despite these differences in perception, both Emily's and Sally's bodies were undergoing similar metamorphoses. In this chapter, I go over some of these basic facts of how a human life begins, before looking in more depth at the foetus's capacities. The growth of the human from an embryo into a foetus, and the journey up until birth, is a complex, almost miraculous process, one in which so much is happening well before the legal age for abortion or the time before which a foetus is considered viable.

Before IVF or surrogacy were available, the only way to conceive was through sexual intercourse – hopefully, but sadly not always, consensual. After a successful conception, we see the start of an extraordinary and very much mutual construction process. The egg that becomes fertilised is initially known as a blastocyst: basically, a ball of fast-dividing cells. This blastocyst releases a hormone (human chorionic gonadotropin, hCG) that instructs the mother's ovaries to stop producing eggs, for the time being at least. It is hCG that can also make the mother nauseous and very sensitive to toxins – as if the tiny nano-being is already protecting itself. This is typical of the complex signalling that takes place constantly, just about all of which is outside the conscious control or awareness of the mother. Many such signals are coming from the foetus, and we might think of these as its survival strategies.

In the first weeks, we see a division of cells into those that will make up the embryo (epiblast) and those that differentiate into the placenta (trophoblast), although in fact miraculously these cells can take on other roles when needed. By about four weeks, this bundle of cells becomes an embryo. It is still a tiny, poppy-seed-sized being, but it has already moved slowly along the fallopian tube and has settled into the extremely nutrient-rich lining of the mother's womb, all the time dividing and growing. From about this time, a test can show if someone is pregnant.

A week later, the now sesame-seed-sized collection of cells already has a flickering heart, the beginnings of a brain, and a hint of other organs such as lungs and intestines. Already the birthgiver's body is changing, and she might feel symptoms, like tiredness, swelling breasts, often needing to go to the toilet, and sometimes a form of spotting that is generally nothing to worry about.

And, of course, many women are assailed by unexpected food attractions or aversions, from pickles to chocolate to strange combinations such as pulled pork on ice-cream! Dairy is a common one, and, indeed, foetal growth can induce serious calcium depletion. A common explanation is that pregnancy gives rise to hormonal shifts or nutrient deficiencies that the body wants to compensate for.[8] Mel told me:

> *I could not stop eating spicy food, the hotter the better, but that was in the early months mainly. Later, weirdly, it was ice cream, I don't usually eat it, but I just could not get enough!*

Or Valerie:

> *I just had to have grapefruit, and then, weirdly, meat, which I normally avoided, and more weirdly, liver, which I generally hate!*

Or, as Dagmar told me:

> *I just wanted ice cubes, even in restaurants I had to ask for ice! The ice thing was all the way through the pregnancy ... I don't know why but I would be just crunching it with my teeth ...*

Dagmar's ice craving is, perhaps surprisingly, not uncommon and has sometimes been linked to anaemic symptoms, a variant of something called pica – a term used to describe cravings for things not normally seen as food, which, for some includes soap, coal, even chalk: indeed, the list is long. No one is quite sure why this happens. The favoured theory is that it is linked to nutrient deficiencies. One study of nearly 300 pregnant women in Ghana[9] suggested that there is some truth to this, especially in relation to anaemia. The women in the study often craved clay as well as starch and, yes, ice, the craving for which is so common that there is even a word for it, 'pagophagia'!

As the pregnancy continues to progress over the next weeks, we see facial features start to form as well as tiny paddle-like hands and feet appearing; in addition, reminding us of our evolutionary amphibian past, there is a tail, which will soon disappear. All this, and yet the new being is still only the size of a small blueberry. We start to call it a foetus, literally meaning 'young one', by about eight weeks. There is often a lot of excitement about becoming pregnant, but what can be missed by those who might be genuinely pleased for you is that it is by no means always easy!

As BBC presenter India Rakusen told me:

> *Yes, it was really exciting to find I was pregnant, but the first trimester was really tough. I was so very tired and felt sick all the time. I was never actually sick, but just really exhausted. I remember in that first trimester calling one of my friends to tell her I was pregnant, and I actually felt quite down and unwell and really struggling to connect, and she was being so excited for me. In fact, I just had to leave the conversation: it was overwhelming for me that someone else could feel all that joy that I was unable to access.*

A similar story was told to me by a psychotherapist, Claire, about when she was in the early stages of her pregnancy:

> *I've realised that as well as the morning sickness making the pregnancy feel hard, I've also been feeling isolated; my partner works away, and this week between away jobs has Covid, so hasn't been able to come home. That is compounded by lots of my closest friends being women who are older than me and not having children but wanting them, and so pregnancy is a very sensitive thing for them, which feels awkward, and to start with I decided not to tell them. That was hard, as I was not feeling my best, being exhausted, having little desire for normal food, and feeling sick.*

Often the feelings at the start of a pregnancy are quite complex, and many women talked about an expectation in others, and in themselves to sound as if everything was sunny and blissful. Several said what a relief it was to be able to share their mixed feelings with others who had been through this. Looking sunny for everyone else is a burden that women do not need!

While the mother is undergoing all these physical and emotional changes, the foetus is doing its own thing, oblivious to its mother's plight. In fact, by 10 weeks the little foetus is quite well formed, its skin still translucent but now with arms and legs that can already move, and even tiny nails starting to form. By now we already see thumb-sucking, and in the next few weeks the little being can kick, stretch, and even hiccough, even if it is still only the size of a fig!

The first trimester finishes at about 13 weeks. That, of course, is when the worst symptoms often abate. Already we see organs, and tiny fingerprints, and, amazingly, this peapod-sized being will, if female, already have ovaries containing several million eggs. It is worth remembering both how well-formed, but also how vulnerable this tiny organism already is, and we will think later about the risks it faces as well as the extraordinary capacities it has.

Most pregnant women breathe a sigh of relief at reaching the second trimester, as from now on the chances of miscarriage reduce dramatically. In fact, many women understandably keep some distance from emotionally attaching too much to the foetus for the first three months, as they cannot be sure the baby won't be lost. Indeed, about one in four foetuses does not make it that far. By the second trimester, the chances of survival increase massively, and, at the same time, with luck, energy ramps up and fatigue reduces. Many women feel especially good at this stage; they are even described as blooming, for example, their hair and skin looking wonderful, and now people notice that they are pregnant. However, as always, there are exceptions. As Gemma told me:

> *I was expecting the second trimester to be all rosy and easy, that's what people told me to expect, but in fact it was a bit of a nightmare. For a start, my sickness carried on much longer than I expected. Worse, I had several episodes of bleeding and felt terrified that my long-awaited baby might not make it. But, worst of all, I had what I only realised later were symptoms of pre-eclampsia, which meant that I often had headaches, my vision seemed all off, and I had stomach pains; I spent a lot of time in bed, just being still. It was all worth it, when my lovely baby arrived, but I felt I missed out on many of the joys of pregnancy.*

Thankfully, Gemma's experiences are uncommon, and many of the women I spoke to said they had never felt so healthy as in the middle trimester, and that they had loved this period.

By 14 weeks, the foetus already has a strong heartbeat, and its internal organs are formed, as are hair, eyelashes, and other features. Indeed, the foetal brain is by now firing away, and it can use facial muscles, move its tongue, as well as swallow. It is soon after this that the biological sex (not gender) of the child can be revealed – something that in nearly all cases is determined by whether the foetus has two X chromosomes or an X and a Y, although there are rare exceptions to this. By around 15 weeks, the apple-sized foetus is actively moving around, and even though its eyes are not yet open, it can, for example, deliberately move away from stimuli like a beam of light. By 16 weeks, male foetuses can start to have erections too!

In the next few weeks, at around 18 to 20 weeks, limbs are more developed, and the foetus might, for example, flex its arms and legs. Indeed, by just over halfway through the pregnancy, its features are already pretty much like a miniature newborn. By now, it will probably be learning to distinguish sounds, like its mother's voice, it might recognise tastes, and its lungs are starting to function. It is learning what to expect from the world it is now inhabiting and, in that process, is also predicting some of what to expect after birth.

The foetus's inner ear reaches adult size by halfway through a pregnancy, and it can now respond, for example, to the sounds of the mother's cardiovascular system, to her bodily movements, to her eating and drinking and food digestion, as well, of course, as to her voice and breathing. It is perhaps no surprise that heartbeat-like sounds are often calming to new babies. Foetal movements are by now generally being felt by the mother, a moment often called the quickening, which tends to start between 16 and 20 weeks.

The third trimester begins at about 27 weeks, and this is the age at which in many modern cultures a foetus is deemed to be potentially viable, although it is unlikely that, in most of human evolutionary history, foetuses would have survived outside the womb anywhere near as early. In the next few weeks, we might see the ability of the foetus to turn its head, it hopefully is starting to put on some healthy fat, and its nervous system is coming online. It can also stretch, and kick now! It can make melanin, which gives its skin its colour as well as its eyes, which will now be partially open and soon fully so, and so able to detect light. The central nervous system is more online, and so it is starting to manage breathing and body temperature. Red blood cells will be forming, hair growing, and the mother will be noticing increased weight gain.

At the start of the third trimester, there are more prods and pokes, although these will normally decrease due to a lack of room for movement from about 34 weeks onwards, as the baby starts to take up most of the amniotic sac. It can now process many more stimuli and control its own temperature.

By about 37 weeks, the baby is preparing for birth. Its bones are hardening, except for those in the skull, which need to be more malleable to make it through the birth canal, and its head, hopefully, is starting to descend into the mother's pelvis. None of this goes unnoticed by the mother, for whom this can be an unpleasant period.

As Emily said:

> *By now there was an uncomfortable heaviness, as I carried around this extra person and their apparatus. My organs were squished, the toilet was a new constant companion, and meals gave way to grazing. This was somewhat tempered by a growing reassurance that all was going ok, something that tentatively increased with every developmental marker of the pregnancy.*

As the foetus is preparing to be born, its own agency increases. I use such language of choice deliberately. The foetus is active and is, in many ways, in charge of much of its destiny, as well, of course, as being utterly dependent – hence the potential of prenatal bonding, which I soon discuss. For much of the pregnancy the foetus is moving, stretching, even tumbling, but as it nears birth, it tends to stay in one position, the hoped-for position generally being head and face down, ready to come through the birth canal. In fact, there are multiple variations, including face up, sideways (transverse), or breach. We hear more details about the birth process itself nearer the end of the book.

What does the foetus get up to?
It's a little being with its own agenda

We have looked briefly at the journey of the foetus, but now I want to think more about how the foetus acts as an autonomous being. Every foetus is both subject and object, influencer and influenced, and is exposed to a huge variety of stimuli. Each foetus develops inside a particular pregnant person, has specific genetic – indeed intergenerational – inheritances, and lives in a unique intrauterine environment. The placenta provides a protective barrier, but many things cross it into the foetus's bloodstream via the umbilical cord, including nutrients, oxygen, of course, but also drugs, alcohol, and various mood-related neurochemicals produced by the mother.

Thus, the foetus is both an utterly dependent creature but also its own being, with its own rhythms, urges, and biological expectations. Its arrival partly transforms the mother's body into the foetus's host. Once plugged into the uterine wall, this tiny being might be said to change its mother's control mechanisms; indeed, some have described this as a bit like how a cosmonaut is really in charge of a spacecraft. The foetus determines how it will lie in pregnancy, which way it will present for the birth, and even the timing of birth. It has feeling and, for example, responds to painful stimuli by turning away, and it demonstrates a surprising capacity for choice. It can actively seek food; indeed, as early as 1937, experiments[10] showed that when saccharin was added to the amniotic fluid, foetuses swallowed more, whereas their drinking rates crashed after the injection of bitter substances.

Some mothers in this phase do, of course, have a range of uncomfortable feelings and realise the indisputable truth: that their bodies are no longer completely their own, that this really is co-embodiment. They might feel nauseous, sick, have strange food desires, as well as swollen breasts and cramps. One mother, Sian, said:

> *I didn't believe I was pregnant, I felt premenstrual and had cramps like when my period is about to start. I felt very uncomfortable, and no one had warned me that this is what can happen. She was already actively being herself before I had any idea that she was even a thing.*

Human learning starts young. Foetuses can soon get used to what at first are unsettling triggers, and, for example, on first encountering a vibrational stimulus placed on the mother's stomach, they might initially move as if disturbed by it, but on subsequent occasions, after they realise it is not a danger, they tend to pay it less attention – an example of a form of learning that psychologists call habituation. Rather than being an inert cell collection, a foetus is active and responsive and is constantly acquiring information that might prove useful.

The foetus is, nonetheless, profoundly influenced by the environment it finds itself in. It can respond to musical signals, moving its limbs in synchrony with musical rhythms.[11] Body movements start at about eight weeks, a few weeks after, a clear heartbeat can be discerned in what is still only a tiny, 5- to 12-millimetre being. In scans we can amazingly see the foetus make facial expressions in active response to music by only 16 weeks.[12] From 10 weeks we can already see movements of the whole body, or at least of a combination of limbs. From 14 weeks on, the mother will probably feel the foetus start to push up against the abdominal wall.[13]

The foetus is not only responding to outside stimuli but has its own rhythms and seemingly does a lot of its own decision making – for example, sometimes opting to swim in the amniotic cavity and at other times resting, all this by the second trimester. Yet outside influences, including the parent's state of mind, can affect the foetus. For example, high levels of stress in the parent will increase foetal movements, even leading to what looks like hyperactivity. Nicotine intake will slow movement, as indeed does diabetes, and, not surprisingly, alcohol also suppresses movement, while cocaine speeds it up. Foetal breathing rates increase after glucose intake and reduce when a mother is fasting, but also, more worryingly, when a mother takes morphine, methadone, or alcohol. The foetus is highly responsive.

As early as the first trimester, the foetus will startle in response to a stimulus placed on a mother's stomach and turn away from a doctor's foetal stethoscope.[14] Foetal heart rates increase when pregnant mothers smoke cigarettes[15] – this is not just immediate reactivity, as the after-effects of maternal smoking can last well into childhood.[16] Ultrasound images have shown foetuses responding both to a mother's cigarette smoking and to external loud noises by what looks on scans very much like crying.[17] Such 4D scans during the last trimester show not only crying and what seems like disgust, but, I am glad to report, also positive states, such as smiling. The foetus will already blink if exposed to a bright light, and by near the end of the pregnancy, the eyes are clearly linked to frontal cerebral areas.

Already we can see the beginnings of nature-nurture interaction: the foetus is both its own being but is also already being socialised. It learns to recognise sounds that it will prefer after birth,[18] particularly the mother's and also, to a lesser extent, the father's or other important adult voices. Culturally influenced tastes are also being picked up, so that, for example, if the mother eats garlic during pregnancy, the newborn will likely show less aversion to it.[19] Incredibly, the foetus shows what seem like innate food preferences, and some health-concerned parents might not be pleased to learn that ultrasound scans show foetuses making smiling-like faces when the mother feeds on carrots but faces more like disgust or a grimace when exposed to kale![20] Each foetus will have its own preferences but will also be influenced by what it is exposed to, and this can affect postnatal taste preferences.

The foetus, as previously described, also influences a mother's food preferences, as Sally shows:

> *I had been a vegetarian for five years, and then, at about 6 months pregnant, I had a sudden demand (it went beyond an urge) for tuna fish. I threw a coat over my pyjamas to rush out to buy some and ate it standing up, straight from the tin. He knew what he needed!*

Foetuses do indeed seem to know what they need. I laughed on hearing my psychiatrist friend Emily's craving for 'quail's eggs and celery salt!' which betrays her class origins, but quails' eggs have larger than average yolks and are a particularly good source of protein, and her baby knew how to get its needs met!

Once the diaphragm has formed, by about 10 weeks, we see more movement and breathing, and, interestingly, even the onset of hiccoughs, which seems to reduce in the last few months of gestation. In fact, for some reason, hiccoughs actually precede breathing by a few weeks.

The foetus is making swallowing movements by 14 weeks, and scans clearly show regular jaw opening and closing. The baby will be taking in amniotic fluid, the fluid that surrounds it. In fact, the baby is often described as being in an amniotic sac. The amniotic fluid also contains a range of nutrients as well as antibodies that help to fight off infection. The sucking and swallowing of amniotic fluid greatly increase by the third trimester.

The pregnant person's state of mind has an impact on the developing foetus. When a sound stimulus is placed against a pregnant mother's stomach, ultrasound scans reveal higher heart rates in foetuses of more depressed mothers than of non-depressed ones. Afterwards, foetuses whose mothers were not depressed or anxious would calm down more quickly than the foetuses of depressed mothers.[21,22] This is uncannily like chronically anxious or stressed older children and, indeed, adults, who tend to have elevated heart rates, something which is often linked to stress; such people also tend to recover more slowly after alarming stimuli. I am certainly one of those. This research suggests that there is already clear prenatal adaptation, and the foetus is preparing for the life it is learning to expect, which might be stress-inducing or calm. This is an important reason for professionals to double-up, at this time, on support for mothers and for mothers to seek support, as such help has been shown to make a big long-term difference.[23]

There remains much still to learn about foetal movements and their significance, but we do know that the kind of movements a foetus makes can be correlated with the integrity of its nervous system. For example, more synchrony in movements of heart rate, eyes, and body predict better capacity for self-regulation and effortful control after birth. In fact, amazingly, it predicts these things right up until adolescence.[13] On the other hand, asynchrony can alert us to the possibility of some issues postnatally. Such issues can be of genetic origin or may be linked to, for example, maternal intake of corticosteroids or alcohol, but either way we can help before and after birth. Brisk, jerky, or hyperactive movements tend to be related to foetal distress, whereas slower than usual movements might be affected by factors like maternal medications. These need not be a cause of alarm but are worth keeping a gentle eye on.

So, the foetus is active, moving, interacting, and not just lying blissfully still in what is probably wrongly called the foetal position. In fact, there is no single foetal position, as foetuses are often changing position, moving their limbs, and might go from supine to sitting to upright or upside down quickly. In their last intrauterine months, they have been seen to raise their hands and place them behind their heads in a seemingly hyper-relaxed style, and even cross their legs as if relaxing in a swing-chair. It would be hard to argue that they were not already, in effect, mini-people, by now acting from a combination of their inherited capacities and responses to their specific intrauterine environment.

CHAPTER 3

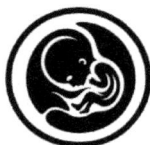

OBSERVING THE UNBORN BABY

With the advent of ultrasound technology, we have gained a never-before-seen window on foetal life. We see foetuses yawn, move about, grimace with pain, undergo rapid eye movement (REM) sleep, and react to noises. By 12 weeks, a foetus will grasp when its palm is stroked, suck when its lips are stimulated, and squint when its eyelids are touched, all of which are observable using 4D scans. Certainly, by about 20 weeks we see a surprising capacity for movement, including crossing legs, swallowing, urinating, and eye movements.

Scans have thus made a big difference to both what we can learn about the unborn child and how we feel about babies. Scans, not surprisingly, pick up much movement that even sensitive mothers do not sense. Of course, what scans pick up is purely visual, and we know how important other senses are in life, especially in the womb. The foetus lives in a world rich in sounds, such as of the heartbeat. Many an unsettled newborn baby is calmed by the sounds familiar to it from before birth, such as of the mother's body sounds as well as rhymes and stories heard while in the womb.

Yet scans have opened up incredible new worlds and insights. Dr Allessandra Piontelli, the pioneer of such work[24] is an Italian psychiatrist who adapted a method of infant observation originally developed in the 1940s at the Tavistock Clinic in London by Esther Bick.[25] I, like many psychotherapy trainees, undertook a weekly hour-long observation of babies, and later I taught this method for years. Piontelli adapted the methodology to observe the foetus with ultrasound for one hour a week from 16 weeks until birth, and she then continued her weekly observations for the first year of the child's life. On reading her work, it becomes evident that each foetus is very much its own person, with a clear personality, one who initiates movements and has preferred positions and ways of being well before birth.

> *One pair of twins, whom she called Marco and Delia, were dizygotic – that is, non-identical. Marco was a passive, inactive foetus, who liked to bury his head in the placental pillow, while his sister was constantly trying out new movements. When she tried to reach out to him in utero, he withdrew; amazingly, this was also the pattern that emerged after they were born. Delia was also much more alert after birth than her brother, who liked to sleep and lie still, just as he had while in the womb.*

In another example, a pair of identical twins, who shared not only the exact same genome but had the rare experience of also sharing the same amniotic sac, were clearly quite different in personality. Possibly surprisingly, the breathing and movements of even identical twins are not necessarily very coordinated.

> *One twin, Giorgio, would move more and earlier than his brother, Fabrizio, and this difference was again seen after they were born.*

This is typical of the many examples Piontelli gives, which suggest that prenatal characteristics persist well into childhood and beyond; we have to wonder whether or not this is an example of innate character.

Whether nature or nurture, such careful observations have allowed us to witness what looks like personalities forming *in utero*. In another pair, a twin who was seemingly more placid and conciliatory *in utero* showed similarly appeasing behaviour with its more aggressive twin in later childhood.

In another touching example:

> *Piontelli had observed through scans a pair of twins being affectionate and stroking each other's heads through a membrane. In their first year after birth, she visited the home and was amazed to see how they stroked each other similarly, but now through a curtain rather than a membrane.*

Less nice to see was a set of twins who were both violent in the womb, seemingly hitting out at each other, and these interaction patterns also persevered as they grew older. Was this just due to the twins' temperament? Or was the intrauterine environment affected by the mother's or family's emotional state, such as stress or anger, and the accompanying release of hormones that cross the placenta? We cannot know for sure, although in this case, the mother was indeed very stressed, through no fault of her own.

Piontelli's accounts may seem anecdotal and open to interpretation, but they suggest that at least some aspects of personality are developing well before birth. As ever, nature and nurture, physiology and psychology, are hard to disentangle. Certainly, her research asks important questions. It might well be that, perhaps unexpectedly, the intrauterine environment is quite different for each twin in a pair. One of them might, for example, claim more space and resources, growing at the expense of the other. Twins clearly do not have identical environments before birth, despite what some longitudinal twin studies assume.

As Anne told me:

> *We were so excited and more than a little stunned to be having twins. It was a monochorionic, diamniotic pregnancy, meaning that there was a shared placenta, but they were in separate sacs. This meant we knew we'd be having identical twins – either two boys or two girls – but did not have to worry about the additional risks that come with monoamniotic pregnancies. There were risks, however, with sharing the placenta, the main one being twin-to-twin transfusion syndrome. This meant we had to have frequent scans, every 2–4 weeks, to check that both babies were developing evenly. Again, I remember frequently praying that the babies would share their space well, and that both would grow at the same rate. I felt anxious before each scan, but at each one we were reassured that they were doing well. Despite these anxieties, I felt so lucky and special to be carrying twins. I can remember exactly where I was when I felt the first kicks, at 17 weeks. At the 20-week scan we decided to find out the sex of the babies, learning that they were girls, which had been my hunch. I found the prospect of having girls to be reassuring. Several close males in my family had serious mental health problems, so I feared that I would worry more about this if I had a son than if I had a daughter.*

Here is a final, sadder example of the effects of prenatal life described by Piontelli:

An 18-month-old baby seemed to be endlessly searching for
something, almost obsessively. The parents reported that this
baby had all along seemed to be acting as if it was looking for
a missing thing and was constantly picking up objects and
shaking them as if to bring them to life. When Piontelli pointed
out that their son seemed to have lost something very important,
the child quietened, and the parents burst into tears, as they told
Piontelli that there had been a twin who had died two weeks
before the birth. The alive twin, who was shaking lifeless objects
and seemed to be desperately looking for something, had spent
two weeks with a dead, unresponsive twin. This intervention
allowed a mourning process to take place in the parents. It also
accelerated Piontelli's longstanding interest in the close bonds so
often seen between twins.

We should remember that far more people lose a twin *in utero* than was once presumed.[26] There is some uncertainty about the extent to which this does or does not leave a lasting mark on the personality, especially given how early on in pregnancies this usually happens. It has been estimated that in around 40% of pregnancies[27] one twin might not survive past the first trimester. The kind of later deaths Piontelli described are thankfully rarer.

Piontelli was probably the first to do such a detailed study of the foetus using ultrasound, and her work continues to make fascinating reading, although these days, with 4D scans and other technology, a much more sophisticated view of the minutiae of foetal development is available, including of the developing brain, which we look at in chapter 4.

CHAPTER 4

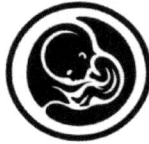

THE DEVELOPING PRENATAL BRAIN: AN AMAZING TRANSFORMATION

During pregnancy, the foetal brain undergoes astonishing growth and maturation, especially in the last trimester. Foetal life is a critical developmental window that can set the stage for brain functioning throughout the lifespan.

In fact, the brain begins to take shape just weeks after conception. Early on, there is just a tiny 3-millimetre neural tube, which then starts its journey to becoming the most complex organ in the known universe – one that has roughly 100 billion neurons at birth. In this process we see extraordinary growth and change, the brain growing as many as up to 15,000,000 nerve cells every single hour! The neural tube is a kind of precursor to the nervous system, transforming in time into the brain and spinal cord.

By just 6 weeks' gestation, major regions like the forebrain, midbrain, and hindbrain are already present. These contain the foundations for structures including the cerebrum, the largest part of the brain, which controls things like movement, as well as the cerebellum, which is small but in fact holds half of all of our neurons and is central for much brain activity, including many emotional responses. Also strongly developing, at the bottom of the brain, is the brain stem, which is connected to the spinal cord and sends messages to the rest of our body. All these vital areas are developing very early in pregnancy and hence are vulnerable to unhealthy influences.

Many things can get in the way of healthy growth, including x-ray exposure, high levels of alcohol, some drugs, as well as some infections, such as German measles (rubella). Professionals and most women are now well aware that throughout pregnancy, and especially during the early stages, good nutrition, avoiding toxins, a generally healthy lifestyle, and, very importantly, minimising too much stress, all improve the chances of optimal brain development. Interestingly, not all medicines are bad. For example, a too-little-known scientist, Katharina Dalton, found evidence that mothers given extra progesterone in the first trimester of pregnancy for reasons other than preventing miscarriage, such as for headaches, had children who consistently had children with higher IQs than children whose mothers had not taken progesterone.[28]

The period when neurogenesis – the name for the generation of new neurons – is at its peak is between 12 and 24 weeks. Incredibly, about 250,000 to 300,000 neurons are created every single minute – yes, every minute – during these months! Synapses are also forming, which connect neurons into networks that allow early capabilities like reflexes, the sensing of stimuli, and basic movement to form into patterns that are written into brain pathways.

In the second trimester, brain growth continues to explode, and this is also when we see both expansion and specialisation. The cerebrum, mentioned above, divides into separate lobes that have different functions, like movement, touch, and vision. The important cerebral cortex is now also growing rapidly, and, as many know, it is vital for skills like cognition, language, and consciousness, and later for planning, empathy, and much that makes us distinctively human.

Already brain areas that allow the foetus to sense and process stimuli are being set up, and these allow the foetus to become able to make choices. As the cerebellum gets bigger, it can start to regulate important motor functions, such as balance and coordination. The hippocampus, which is crucial for memory formation and spatial navigation, also matures. Thus, by only 20 weeks, all the infrastructure is in place for the trillions of connections that enable the newborn's amazing capacities.

Yet, while overall brain architecture is complete by mid-pregnancy, in the third trimester we see important and rapid development involving extensive rewiring, which strengthens and refines connections between neurons. Dendrites, which look like little tree branches at the end of neurons, sprout and enable efficient communication between cells. At the same time, we see what is called synaptic pruning, the deliberate loss of cells that are not needed, which means that pathways that survive are honed into efficient circuits. By now we see the start of the development of what is called grey matter in the outer cerebral layers. We also see the formation of white matter via the process of myelination, myelin being the fatty sheath that insulates axons and dramatically speeds communication between cells. The foetal brain is also clearly emitting brain waves by the seventh month.

The prefrontal cortex continues to mature, and this will, in time, support vital executive functions like focus, reasoning, and impulse control, while REM sleep patterns are emerging now as the foetus alternates between wakeful and sleeping states. By 37 weeks, this intricate organ is primed for life after birth.

Despite its remarkable transformation, the tiny foetal brain is very vulnerable. Occasionally bad luck occurs, such as in rare pregnancies where the neural tube may fail to close properly, resulting in defects like spina bifida, a condition that can now be operated on *in utero*. Some kinds of infections can damage the developing nervous system. Most importantly, the more we enhance a mother's physical and mental health, the lower is the risk of any neurodevelopmental issues. Very high stress-hormone exposure (and I mean very high, not the kind we might expect to see in normally stressed parents) can impair the growth and survival of neurons. Nutritional deficiencies can also mean that the foetus runs short of important nutrients, especially the proteins, fats, vitamins, and minerals that are essential for optimal brain maturation.

Unfortunately, there is always conflicting nutritional advice on offer. Some research suggests, for example, that a Mediterranean diet aids cognitive development[29]. David Barker,[30] the foremost researcher on foetal programming whose work I describe in chapter 9, warned of many dangers of poor nutrition, such as low birth weight. This is a subject that is still being researched.[31] The current consensus, which can, of course, change, is that consuming a nutrient-rich prenatal diet, which includes choline, folate, iron, fatty acids, and antioxidants, is likely to foster healthy brain maturation.

Alcohol, at least more than a small amount, can be damaging to the vulnerable foetal brain, as we will hear more about. Other substances, like nicotine, opioids, and cocaine, can also cross the placenta into foetal circulation, where they interfere with neurotransmitters and brain-signalling pathways.

Perhaps still underestimated and too little understood, environmental toxins like lead and mercury are starting to be shown to adversely influence brain development. I hesitated to write this, as there is so much out of our control, but perhaps it is worth knowing that, for example, microplastics have been discovered in placentas during pregnancies, and these can contain endocrine disruptors.[32] Some people have even linked this phenomenon with the increase in autistic spectrum traits, but this relationship is certainly as yet unproven.[33]

Because foetal brains develop so rapidly, this tiny window of development is of vital importance. Treating infections early, avoiding harmful substances and stress, where possible, will protect the developing nervous system. Regular exercise, social support, and stress reduction will benefit both mother and child. Above all, providing expectant mothers with the resources for a healthy pregnancy allows infants' brains to start life with the best possible neural foundation. Well before birth, many factors can affect the future human for better or worse, and we can consciously make a big difference to the outcomes. More of this in later chapters.

CHAPTER 5

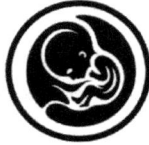

WOW OR WOO:
INTERACTING AND BONDING
WITH THE UNBORN BABY

B onding and becoming close to one's unborn baby can
take many forms. Sally told me:

> *I had literally no life plan at that stage – an unhappy marriage*
> *and being sacked from my training as a nurse because I was*
> *pregnant. My husband was unreliable, and we had no financial*
> *security at all. It was a scary time. But I was in love! In love*
> *with my son. I just knew he was a boy, and I felt such a*
> *powerful yearning for him throughout my pregnancy. I also lost*
> *any remaining interest in my husband, I just longed for my son.*
> *I didn't go to any antenatal groups, I didn't know they existed,*
> *I was just in a sort of trance.*

Prenatal bonding has become something of a trend in the
last few years. Some claims for it might, at the outset, seem a
bit leftfield, even 'woo', but in fact much of the research is

very promising. However, we should remember that such bonding does not always happen. I worked for many years with children in the social care system who had experienced trauma in the family. One adolescent, whom I call Jemma, reported to me that she felt upset when she found she was pregnant and did not want to keep her baby. She said:

> *I was angry with my boyfriend and 'ditched him'. I wanted to have the baby adopted because I didn't like the idea of an abortion. But at about three or four months it changed. I don't know why. I think it was seeing the scan and then feeling it start to move around. It felt weird, but I knew I definitely wanted to keep her, yes, a she, and that feeling just grew. I was scared, but I wanted this more than anything I ever had before. It was the best decision I ever made.'*

The best known early work on prenatal bonding was conducted by the Hungarian psychoanalytic practitioner, Jenő Raffai,[34] who had impressive results, even if his explanations of how this happened can be debated. He collected data from over 4,300 pregnant women who used what he described as prenatal bonding techniques. The reported benefits seem extraordinary. The mothers in his programmes experienced less pain and anxiety during labour; the labours were less complicated, with fewer obstetric interventions and with very low levels of birth trauma. What is often called 'excessive infant crying' after birth was almost unknown in this group. Another huge boon to parents who used these methods was that their babies slept longer and deeper at night. Incredibly, postpartum depression was less than 1%, which is very much less than the usual 10% to 15% often quoted. Where there was a father or another parental figure in the picture, the results got even better. When a couple jointly tries to bond with their unborn baby, then this often strengthens the bond between the couple too, which has its own positive knock-on effects on the baby. Indeed, Dutch attachment-informed researchers have recently started hopeful-looking experiments with fathers using ultrasound to enhance prenatal paternal bonding.[35] While it is true that Raffai had a somewhat self-selecting sample, nonetheless there seem to be important lessons to be taken from his work.

The concept of bonding has been misused by many psychologists and attachment-informed people, as there has been a longstanding misconception that bonding must occur immediately after birth, otherwise irrevocable damage can occur. This is an idea that was popularised in the 1960s and 1970s through animal studies. For example, greylag geese will follow around the first creature of any species that they see, and sheep will imprint on their lambs' smells and reject advances from lambs lacking the right scent. Humans are different, though, and we do not have a critical period straight after, let alone before, birth when bonding must occur. Human adults have the potential to bond with most babies, not just their own, and such bonding rarely happens immediately; rather, it takes time to develop. John Bowlby,[36] the founder of attachment theory, found that it is consistent care and closeness over time that gives rise to what he termed 'affectional' (meaning emotional, not necessarily affectionate) bonds. Affectional, or emotional, bonds between a mother and a foetus can, it seems, form well before birth, but, if they don't, there is time for this to happen later.

Bowlby's attachment theory is now very well-known and has mostly stood up over time. I remain proud to have worked for several decades at the Tavistock, where Bowlby bravely developed his incredible theories. However, one thing Bowlby was wrong about was that he thought humans were like many other mammals where there is instant one-to-one bonding. We now know that humans are unlike most other primates and mammals in that we are what is unflatteringly called a 'co-operative breeding species'.[37] We, in our evolutionary history, have reared our young in groups and almost never in nuclear families. In other words, until recently there were many more adults involved in bringing up a child than we see now in our modern-day, evolutionarily unusual, and often emotionally challenging single-dwelling family set-ups. This is one major reason why contemporary parenting is such a tough challenge.

We live in an individualistic culture and tend to assume that babies and children inevitably live in nuclear families. This has rarely been the case in human evolutionary history; we evolved to live in multi-family groups, and babies evolved to have many adults around them. In fact, I would suggest that the more we can foster such multiple-adult caretaking systems with alternative or additional caregivers, the more emotionally healthy is the baby – and, indeed, also the parents. Developmental psychologist and psychoanalyst Ed Tronik[38] studied a hunter-gatherer group called the Efe and found that babies tended to spend less than 50% of their time being cared for by their mothers; they could be passed to well over a dozen adults in the average hour. They still had primary attachment figures, such as their mothers, fathers, and grandparents, but they learnt that it was safe reassuring and enjoyable to be cared for by multiple adults in the close-knit groups they lived in.

Important in such societies is the idea that a baby is not the property of an individual set of parents but is part of a culture, of a wider community, and, indeed, is a representative of an ancestral history. The Navajo, for example, saw pregnancy as a time to connect past, present, and future generations. In many such cultures, elders and the whole community have traditionally been involved. Often there are rituals connecting with time-honoured traditions, ways of linking the birthgiver and the unborn child to the community and culture. Typical is how, in Kenya, Maasai fathers undertake various rites during pregnancy, including constructing a special hut for the birth. Again, we should not glamorise such cultures' approach to pregnancy and birth. The Maasai, for example, have very high infant mortality and high rates of sexual violence, and they have traditionally practiced female genital mutilation, but hopefully we can still learn from their emphasis on community life and ancestral traditions.

Returning to bonding, if we take it to mean the development of a close relationship in which people are in some way psychologically and emotionally 'bonded' together, then we can see how this might happen in prenatal life. Indeed, some of Bowlby's psychoanalytic contemporaries, such as Therese Benedek[39] and Helen Deutsch,[40] were by the middle of the twentieth century finding that, as a pregnancy moves forward, the foetus often becomes more loved and is also experienced increasingly as a separate being, not just an extension of the mother.

During the 1960s, Reva Rubin and others suggested that what we were seeing in many mothers was prenatal attachment. She suggested that as such attachments form, there is a change of mindset, so that the mother becomes concerned with tasks such as ensuring safe passage of the foetus, or that the unborn child will be accepted by significant others in the mother's life. Some readers will recognise this shift. Such an emotional attachment includes, for example, a desire to sacrifice her own wishes for the baby. Rubin wrote:

> *By the end of the second trimester, the pregnant woman becomes so aware of the child within her and attaches so much value to*

him that she possesses something very dear, very important to
her, something that gives her considerable pleasure and pride .[41]

This, of course, will not be news to most pregnant women, but such early research captured what perhaps women knew and most men did not: that the foetus is, by midway through the pregnancy, thought of as a real person with whom mothers had a 'real relationship in their imagination'.[42] Interestingly, Ruben found that the earlier this was established, the fewer the problems seen later, and that lack of such an imaginative caring bond was often indicative of factors such as a lack of interest or support by partners and family. This might fit with research that shows clearly that when there is good prenatal bonding, generally there is also good postnatal bonding,[43] or in other words, that the good feelings and relationships from before birth continue afterwards.

There is debate about whether what these researchers are describing should be called 'attachment', but they certainly are describing ways in which a birthgiver is forming a relationship with the unborn baby, not only in body, but also in heart and mind. These early researchers showed what is often missed in accounts of foetal behaviour: that even at this stage there can be love, care, and the ability to imagine the life of the unborn child.

One of the original terms used to describe this was mother–foetal attachment (MFA),[44] but, of course, fathers and other caregivers, as well as parents who are trans men, can also develop their own important bonds with the unborn baby. It might not be bidirectional, in the sense of a foetus being able to attach to and relate as yet to a separate person, but, as John Condon, a researcher from the 1990s, said, the pregnant mother seeks *'to know, to be with, to avoid separation or loss, to protect, and to identify and gratify the needs of her foetus.* [45]

A birthgiver can have both an emotional and a psychological relationship with the foetus, and when this does happen, outcomes tend to be better. It is, again, worth stressing that this is not just about mothers. There has been impressive research on fathers, looking at prenatal paternal attachment. In fact, scales have even been devised to measure how fathers relate to their unborn child, and one could equally devise scales or research measuring prenatal attachment with other caregivers, such as second mothers.

Different meetings: scans and senses

The possibilities for bonding increased greatly when scans of foetuses became part of standard medical practice. It was noticed that after having an ultrasound, just having and looking at such an image seemed to foster an increase in warm feelings towards the unborn baby – a fact that has since been backed up by research.[46] Nowadays, first scans are carried around in handbags or wallets, seen on fridge magnets, and make their way into family photo albums. In fact, it seems that 3D (still image) and 4D (moving image) scans considerably increase good feelings for the foetus, apparently more so in fathers. A 4D scan will show an active foetus making, for example, movements and facial expressions.

One dad, Mick, told me:

> *I was not at all sure I wanted to be a father. In fact, I was quite cross that it had happened, and I was moody and not very nice for a few weeks! I went somewhat unwillingly to the hospital for the first scans, but something really changed when I saw the*

images and I saw this real, alive being, who had come from me, from us, and I felt a sudden warmth, an urge to relate, to be in contact. I knew then that this was what I wanted.

Such 4D scans, which show something clearly alive and active, allow us to believe in the existence of a being who is almost a proper person, who has agency and can interact, and with whom we can imagine having a reciprocal relationship. The parent or involved adult can more easily start to feel warmly towards the unborn child when seeing them express their will, or move with purpose, inside the womb. This is part of what it means to feel bonded with one's unborn child.

One interesting study, though,[47] reported that, while ultrasounds were experienced as helpful by many mothers – in large part because they helped them to really trust that they had an alive baby inside them, something that can lead to initial bonding – there was also a downside. It was found that an over-reliance on scans could inhibit a mother's ability to trust her own senses, to really feel, kinaesthetically, their baby in their body. It is that process of getting to know the baby and connecting psychologically, emotionally, and physiologically that can give rise to a better bonding outcome. So, the scans might be helpful initially, but over-reliance on them can take the mother too far away from her own bodily and emotional experience.

As my doula colleague and yoga teacher Nikita Akilapa said, one of the things pregnant women need more of is trust in their own senses. Instead, all too often they are expected to trust, not their own bodies, but medical expertise and technology, which might be being used for the right motives but can also be disempowering. As she pointed out, women who have more scans might have more medical issues and are often already feeling more fear. She told me:

> *I try and help people understand that body wisdom, which includes sensation, and also instinct, is just as important as medical research because the medical model is based on a generic understanding based on statistics and academic studies, but not on a woman's particular experience in the moment.*

Here is an example from Anne, whose life really changed after her first scan:

> *I remember praying, 'please let me get pregnant with twins in October', having come off the pill in September. Nothing happened in the next few months, but in the following February I did become pregnant. I was excited, but also anxious, as my closest friend had sadly just had a 'missed miscarriage' and found out about it at her 12-week scan. I was driving my husband so potty with my worries about whether I was really pregnant that he agreed for us to get a private scan at nine weeks. In that scan, we learned that there was not one, but two tiny foetuses with healthy heart beats. Now everything really, truly had changed!!*

For other women, it is indeed the bodily experience of the baby inside that makes it all real, as Emily described:

> *The movements within gave something real in the physical realm, at first just a faint fluttering: is that what I think it is? Then later, a dramatic bid for space internally as my little one stretched and stuck out a foot, defying the usual boundaries of my stomach. It is both amusing and terrifying at once.*

One important infancy researcher, Charley Zeanah,[48] found that mothers who scored as having higher levels of prenatal attachment were more likely to perceive and notice foetal movement than those who scored as having a lower level of prenatal attachment. This was linked to them noticing a foetus's capacity for interaction – for example, feeling the foetus moving towards the abdomen when it is stroked, or changing its levels of movement when a familiar voice is heard. The good news is that such awareness can be learnt and developed, such as via prenatal yoga classes. As Nikita said:

> *I really try and help people understand that your body wisdom – which includes sensation, instinct, and intuition – is really important at birthing time. This can help to be vocal with your care team about what you feel, and advocate for what your body is requesting.*

Awareness of one's own bodily signals, often called interoception, can be facilitated and taught, such as in therapy, yoga, and meditation. Sadly, much in our society goes against this, including birth control, pain relief medications, and the ease of getting medical products. Yoga classes have the additional benefit of women learning from other women and seeing how others recognise their sensations, supporting each other in becoming more bodily aware, such as realising that a passing sensation they might not have ordinarily noticed could well, in fact, have some meaning.

So, although prenatal attachment is very different from attachment after birth, what the research convincingly shows[49] is that where there is a good prenatal bond, we tend, after birth, to see better outcomes, such as in feeding behaviour, parental sensitivity to infant cues, and much more.

Given this, it does seem that anything we can do to improve prenatal bonding is going to be a good thing for all. Indeed, the opposite is worryingly true: if prenatal attachments are poor, or if the attachment style of pregnant mothers is insecure, then outcomes can be worse and can lead to less satisfactory relationships after birth.[50] The good thing is that we can help ourselves and others, whether via therapy or informal or formal support systems. Ambivalence and mixed feelings are so much part of life, and especially of parenting, and they need to be acknowledged and accepted, in a sense folded into our experience in a compassionate way. There is quite enough judgement in this space already! There can be tremendous relief in knowing, and allowing, and sharing ambivalence and difficult feelings generally, especially with other pregnant women; and, of course, if the feelings are particularly overwhelming, then more formal support can be helpfully sought.

Actively communicating with the unborn baby

The claims made by Raffai[26] and others about prenatal bonding, and the extraordinarily positive results they have reported, have led to prenatal bonding being researched more thoroughly. Raffai was a psychoanalyst whose clinical work suggested that many of his most disturbed clients could trace their psychological issues back to prenatal life, and hence he came to understand the importance of this period in life. He found in work with his patients what the research shows, that serious events, such as the loss of a birthgiver's partner during pregnancy, can have catastrophic effects on foetal life and growth. Powerful shocks, physical assaults, drugs, and much else will not only affect the mother's body but also the way the foetus develops.

The opposite, thankfully, is also true, and a foetus can respond positively to soothing or enjoyable experiences. Going back several decades, it has been found that a foetus can have a positive response to music and will, for example, move differently to calming music as opposed to hip-hop, its heart rates similarly altering.[51] Moving in rhythm to music, especially if it is soothing, enhances prenatal central nervous system development and has beneficial effects, such as reducing stress.[52] Most important, of course, is the effect on the foetus of a mother's calm and loving state of mind.[53] One mother, my yoga teacher and friend Annabel Chown, told me:

> *I would lie quietly on the sofa and put on my favourite tracks, and I would feel calm, but I just felt that he too would be calm; not still, in fact sometimes I would swear he was moving to the music, but it was as if we were experiencing this together.*
>
> *I wasn't one of those women who did lots to specifically connect with her baby during pregnancy, like play special music to it. But I'd like to think my buoyant mood, my meditation and yoga practice, my endless walks round London, all the great food I ate, all served him well.*

Fascinatingly, it has been found that in the third trimester, and possibly before, when mothers are asked to deliberately communicate with their unborn babies by touching their abdomen and by talking to them, foetuses have a clearly positive reaction, such as indulging in less self-soothing while being touched or opening their mouths when being talked to. Neither reaction occurs with non-communicative talking or touch.[54] True, the foetus picks up stress, via cortisol, by epigenetic dysregulation of the placenta, by inflammation in the mother, or by dysregulation of the microbiome, but it can also pick up positive signals, and this gives rise to the possibility of more hopeful emotional communication from very early on.

For mothers who do want to bond more with their babies – hopefully, the majority – Raffai's work provides many clues. The way Raffai worked was by facilitating a mother to develop mental images of her unborn baby, and to then send silent messages to the baby. This, he suggested, gives rise to a change in the physiological states of both the mother and the baby. In fact, he suggests that the foetus receives messages from the birthgiver and responds accordingly, as if the baby knows it is being talked to and hears what is said. Some wonder whether there is some kind of neuronal communication in which brainwave signals, such as alpha and delta waves, which are also involved in meditative states, are somehow transmitted to the unborn baby. This is speculation, but clearly in such interventions changes do take place in the mother's nervous system and in how a baby is and acts.

As Valerie told me:

> I longed more and more to commune with my child, but this was not easy: a 100-mile daily round commute by car and a full-time teaching job meant my outer life was busy. Stepping into a warm bath in my off time meant that I could let go and really connect with my inner experience. The warm water enveloped me as I pictured my child within my own waters. I longed to not only commune but know more – what exactly was happening, at what stage was my child? What did it look like? I found a battered copy of, 'A Child is Born' and took great comfort in the colour plates of the foetus as it developed. This became a sort of bible for me; bobbing in the warm bath with my baby and using the book to help me visualise its development. It felt reassuring. I could let the day drift away as I turned to, and then let go, of the book to just be with my unborn child in the secure watery warmth.

Therapeutic work to improve prenatal bonding aims to build a relationship between the mother and the foetus. A central aspect of this is to help a mother become aware of the states of being and, indeed, the emotions of the foetus. Such therapeutic work is thus aimed at constructing a bonding space and, we might also say, a mentalising space, to start thinking about the unborn baby as a being with needs and feelings.

In Emily's words:

> *I at times conducted a commentary, silent or otherwise, or sang a song. I read and watched keenly the images of a growing foetus from a book, as mine reached the same stage. But really the most important sense was of a growing presence within, of a growing fantasy of who the little person was. It happened without my design really, but the relationship deepened, embellished, and responded. The movements within made something real in the physical realm, at first just a faint fluttering – is that what I think it is? Then later, a dramatic bid for space internally as my little one stretched and stuck out a foot, defying the usual boundaries of my stomach. It was both amusing and terrifying at once. Would it burst out like an alien? But something had become solid by then, an understanding of our different territories and an acceptance, and most times, a love of this constant companionship.*

The form of therapeutic work facilitated by Raffai and colleagues would be aiming to develop just this kind of insight, I think. It often includes helping the mother to process her own prenatal and birth experiences, which otherwise can get in the way of mentalising and bonding. Parents are often given homework. For example, mothers might be encouraged to sit in a rocking chair and become emotionally present to their baby for ten minutes a day. Rocking is also one of the best-known ways of stimulating the foetus's growing vestibular system, which is central to balance and coordinated movement. Fathers, or other caregivers, can play a role in many ways, such as by stroking the baby through the abdominal wall, singing songs, or reading stories to the foetus.

Much of this is in the service of creating a space for bonding and communication. Obviously, the yet-to-be born baby cannot understand verbal symbols, but the mother can try and 'read' the baby's states and communicate something of emotional significance back. Images are central to Raffai's way of working:

> Raffai describes a case where the baby was presenting for birth in the breech position and the mother, not surprisingly, was fearful of birth complications. She was encouraged to ask the baby to turn around but did not do as suggested. This might have felt like a strange request – certainly, it would be for many mothers. Soon after, though, she made a connection to something important in her own history, which is that she herself had been born breech. After this, she calmed down and was helped to speak inwardly to the baby and let it know that it need not do as she did. Amazingly the baby turned around.

Make of that what you will! Of course, there are other ways of facilitating such communication. Nikita Akilapa explained how she always used the resting pose, Shavasana, at the end of a yoga class as a time for mothers to tune into their babies and their signals and movement; she says that not every mother does this naturally, of course, but that these are definitely skills that can be learnt.

Active birth and yoga teacher Jessica James, who is also a parent–infant and group psychotherapist and, also in fact my/our active birth teacher, told me:

> Through these classes, you can help mothers start to identify more with their babies and learn to be in touch with them. I might say things like, 'You're breathing deeply, when you're getting more oxygen, so are your babies.' 'You're slowing down, you're relaxing, and maybe your babies like it and you can feel

your baby's response in their movements.' I am just bringing the baby subtly, and gently, into the class as a real person. Women may say, 'Oh, my husband talks to our baby', or 'I play music to my baby, and I think my baby likes it, I get kicks'. Hearing about each other's experiences gives ideas. It's a subtle approach, about developing a capacity for attentive care, not about being instructed. A lot can be done just by helping women to get comfortable holding their tummies and experiencing their babies in new ways in a safe space.

This was echoed by India Rakusen:

I'm way more aware of the importance of prenatal bonding this time around, having gone through pregnancy once and had a baby. It's now easier to imagine what prenatal bonding might look and feel like. This time I'm spending less time with my head in books and more time with my hands on my tummy. And, from making programmes about pregnancy and women's bodies, I am so much more aware of him as an alive, separate being, of what he is learning in the womb, what he's taking in. Society and the law and a parent can have completely different perspectives on what this thing is within a womb. There are so many debates about when a foetus is and isn't a human being, but he's like born, a human being, but living in a kind of a case.

There are many stories from traditional cultures that suggest that these kinds of ideas are not all that unusual. For example, the Beng of West Africa[55] believe that babies come from a place of spirits called *wrugbe* and are reincarnations of ancestors. The anthropologist Alma Gottlieb described a Beng woman having a difficult childbirth who summoned a diviner who told her that the baby would only come out when she called the name the baby had had in *wrugbe*. When the mother did this, the anthropologist witnessed that the birth proceeded speedily. In some ways, this sounds rather like some of Raffai's prenatal bonding interventions, except that in the case of the Beng, the diviner's intervention is rooted in a longstanding set of beliefs about a spirit world, and how a new baby is part of an intergenerational set of traditions.

Many other cultures have similar pregnancy rites. In Māori traditions in difficult labours a healer or *tohunga* will often incant a spiritual chant or *karakia* to bring about the birth.

The Hausa in Nigeria use rituals like henna painting and dances that celebrate imminent motherhood. In Zuni Native American culture an elder woman rubs cornmeal over the pregnant woman's belly before birth as a form of blessing. Many non-WEIRD (i.e., not Western educated industrialized rich democratic) cultures have rituals with such a spiritual element. Some of the beliefs might be hard for us WEIRD people to relate to, but what these examples do demonstrate is the sense of the unborn baby as already part of a wider culture and set of beliefs and traditions and a being who already is seen as part of that world and can be communicated with. This is less present in Western approaches to foetal life and birth, and some might think this is a loss.

From a Western psychological lens, there are often powerful unconscious factors that can get in the way of a smooth birthing process. Raffai relates how one mother was reported to have a seemingly inexplicable fear of a premature birth. It turned out that her own mother had been in a hurry to finish the pregnancy and give birth so that she could return to her career. Presumably, the early pregnancy and the subsequent disaster of being abandoned remained with the now-pregnant mother as what is sometimes called a foetus's intrauterine maternal representation.[34] Here is a paraphrase of Raffai's account:

One mother had not planned to get pregnant, and the potential new baby had disrupted many of her life plans. Since learning she was pregnant, she had never consciously shown resentment or a wish to terminate the pregnancy. However, one might wonder if the foetus' dangerously elevated pulse of between 160 and 320 was how such ambivalence showed itself. In the intervention the mother was encouraged to develop an image of a loving hand with which she imagined massaging the baby from head to toe. The foetal pulse rate soon came down to about 160, albeit still too high. She was then encouraged to use an inner voice in which she said 'You have arrived unexpectedly. It has taken us time to accept and love you. You must have felt that we did not want you, this must have been heartbreaking for you. But know that we have accepted you and love you. You are important to us' (p. 68[26]). This gave rise to profuse weeping in the mother during which the foetus too reacted strongly. Yet almost miraculously a while later the pulse rate had lowered to 140.

Again, assuming this anecdote is accurate, we might all have our own explanations of what happened and how and why, but presumably the mother's processing of her own feelings led her to feel more at peace in herself, and that could have been transmitted to the foetus.

Raffai's suggestion is that in such work the foetus understands at some level that it is being thought about and that it is being related to as an alive being with a will and mind and feelings. What is certainly happening is that the mother can be in touch with her own thoughts and emotions – often disowned ones – as well as with her bodily sensations during the pregnancy, and this will have a kind of knock-on effect on her nervous system and also on the intrauterine environment.

Raffai's methods might sound strange to some. In fact, many people feel uneasy just talking to any children, let alone babies – let alone foetuses! Yet, whatever the actual mechanism, the methods can clearly pay dividends. Raffai's accounts describe many mothers who had to let go of their embarrassment and learn how to talk to their foetus. In Raffai's sample, what did not seem to help was more idle chat to the baby, such as a mother describing her day at work. It was only when the foetus is talked to and feels addressed, according to Raffai, that we see changes. The pulse example given above is by no means unique, and, indeed, a decreased foetal pulse rate is common when love is overtly felt by the mother and expressed. It is also worth noting that these babies do not respond to strangers' voices or touch, only the mothers' or other voices of people with whom a bond is developing.

> *In a more medically risky story, a mother and baby had bonded well but in the 36th week her placenta began to deteriorate, and the doctors were considering a caesarean section. The mother was in a panic but, when guided to massage the baby with what Raffai calls her inner mental hand, her test results dramatically improved within a day or two and the caesarean was no longer needed. The placenta somehow regenerated, so a normal birth could take place at the appointed time.*

Friends and colleagues have reported similar things. Perinatal specialist Karina Sarmiento told me of a similar case where birth was late, and the doctors were pressuring for a caesarean section; the mother talked to her unborn baby and invited him to come out naturally. In this case, amazingly, the baby came out of its own accord soon after, and the risk of a caesarean was averted. Nikita Akilapa told me:

> *I always encourage pregnant people to talk to their babies and ask them for whatever it is that's needed. For example, you can tell them you're ready for them to come now, that you're so*

excited to meet them. Or, if they're breech, tell them that you want them to turn. I often use the final resting pose in yoga class for this – I remind everyone that it's a good time to connect with baby, receive any messages they have for you, and share any you have for them.

There are countless other similarly interesting stories from the literature or clinical examples. You, as a reader, need to make up your own mind about them. Raffai, for example, describes a mother making emotional contact with the baby, upon which the baby moved up near her heart. However, when it pressed against the mother's heart, this hurt her, and the mother was then helped to suggest to her baby that it move down a bit. The baby did but then hit the abdomen, which again hurt the mother, who asked it silently to come back up a bit. Guess what, it did! Is this a coincidence?

Whether or not all the stories in this chapter are convincing scientifically, and whether they are more akin to the description of pregnancy and birth by the Beng people described above, what seems clear is that something important and health-enhancing happens in such attempts to interact and emotionally bond with the foetus. With a range of rituals in which the unborn baby is related to and taken seriously – whether with Beng rituals, the pregnancy sash worn by Mongolian women to protect them spiritually (as reported in chapter 6), or the prenatal bonding methods employed by Raffai – something seems to shift in the direction of hope and, indeed, love, and in that process something in the baby changes too.

Understanding about prenatal bonding can make a real material difference to the experience of pregnancy. Claire wrote to me, saying:

Reading the first draft of your book made me realise how possible it was to connect with this tiny embryonic person even at this early stage (6 weeks). I started talking to him in my mind (he feels like a 'he'), lying with my hand over him tuning in, or visualising stroking him with my 'mental hand', as in Raffai's studies. It really shifted my relationship and allowed an emotional connection with him, when before it was just nausea and hope. I'd get a massive craving for a boiled egg and say, 'Oh, you'd like an egg, would you?' Or I'd experience a huge almost panicky hunger and could reassure him that the food was coming and take deep breaths to calm my own system, and his environment, while a potato cooked in the microwave. Even when I get sick now, I think, 'Ah, you want me to rest more, do you? Are you not getting enough of my resources as I'm rushing around? I'll see what I can do.' It's lovely to think that already this proto-person is learning that the world and I care about his needs and want to listen to him and help him cope with difficult things. And that when he's born, we'll already have established a trusting, collaborative relationship.

When I next heard from Claire, I learnt that not only was all well with the pregnancy but also that, as her intuition picked up, she was indeed carrying a boy!

CHAPTER 6

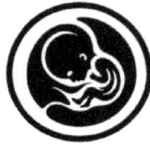

CULTURE AND INDIGENOUS KNOWLEDGE

M ost of this guide is based on research with Western samples, from people in so-called WEIRD societies, and so it does have a clear bias. I am imagining that many but certainly not all readers fit into this cultural category too, although many of us have our origins in very different cultures and traditions. I have always believed that it is vital that we learn as much as we can from and about other cultures and their practices. For one thing, it makes us less prejudiced, and less certain that we have all the answers. This is especially important at a time when we are increasingly aware of the pernicious effects of colonialism and prejudice.

In addition, what we call 'modern' societies have not been in existence for very long, at most a few thousand years, and modern capitalist economies only a few hundred years. Yet our bodies, brains, and nervous systems evolved over millions of years and have not changed much in the last few thousand. In making sense of prenatal life and what it is important to be aware of, there can be a place for both science and ancestral wisdom. In fact, many parents I speak to feel that contemporary family life, based around nuclear families and the commodification of childhood, is missing important elements of meaning that other cultures have historically valued, and which could possibly be reclaimed in some ways.

We live in a particularly individualistic society in which health-enhancing social ties have been thinning for decades.[56] The rise of depression and loneliness has been linked to this;[57] indeed, this is so serious that the World Health Organization declared loneliness a serious health epidemic. Historically, most cultures have seen pregnancy and birth as part of a journey in which history, ancestry, spiritual beliefs, and social cohesion are central. For example, in Māori culture, there is a belief that infants are linked to ancestors and a spiritual realm. Indeed, they have a ritual called Oriori, in which each child receives their own personalised lullaby, which helps guide them through their own specific challenges and their life journey. This is different to modern science's view that processes such as birth are purely biological ones that only need skilled technicians and not any ancestral wisdom. Something important about cultural transmission has been lost. No new human life is really a new life: there are always cultural, biological, and familial histories and traditions, and birth – like death – is a rite that can benefit from having ceremony and a sense of awe about it.

In most cultures studied, anthropologists have found specific rituals designed to protect both mother and baby during pregnancy. In Mongolian nomadic culture, for example, pregnant women wear a pregnancy sash that provides spiritual protection; in fact, these women often have strong pregnancies and ride their horses right up until birth! By the same token, the Ndebele people of Zimbabwe avoid verbally praising a pregnant woman to avoid attracting negative spirits, a bit like the idea of the evil eye seen in many societies such as Turkey's. The Beng of Ivory Coast discourage pregnant women from handling monkey meat, to avoid babies being born with deformities. Such practices are a culture's way of making meaning of this potent life transition and maintaining the health of the mother and baby.

Many cultures have rich symbolic rituals and belief systems around fertility, conception, pregnancy, and birth. Some rituals aim to protect against dangerous spirit forces. The Dagara people of Burkina Faso do not allow a pregnant woman to walk at night, as this is seen as risky; similarly, the Cuna of Panama prohibit pregnant women from walking at noon, when evil spirits are active. The Ewe of West Africa have mothers wear a girdle of charms and amulets. Igbo tribesmen of Nigeria have supervised ritual points of transition like the quickening, while Curanderos, traditional Mesoamerican healers, used prayer and herbal baths to spiritually cleanse Aztec pregnant women. These are all signs of an awareness of how vulnerable the foetus and mother are during this period and how in need of protection, in part by time-honoured rituals.

There are non-science-based beliefs and practices in WEIRD cultures too, such as how some believe it is unlucky to buy gifts for a baby before it is born, or that it also is risky to tell people about a pregnancy before the end of the first trimester. There will be other rituals we might not even be aware of. Some believe that if a mother raises her arms above her head, this might risk the umbilical cord doing damage, which, as you might imagine, has no evidence; others, including people of my own heritage, discourage attendance at funerals, believing that ghosts and ghouls may badly affect the unborn baby – although it is probably true that strain and upset on the part of the mother are not good for the foetus. So-called superstitions in the contemporary world are probably much more widespread than we care to admit – for example, how many pregnant women consider it bad luck to walk under a ladder?

In many cultures, pregnancy divination is used to determine the unborn child's sex, analyse omens for birth, and detect supernatural causes of complications. Of course, it is not uncommon for pregnant women in Eurocentric cultures to have their fortune read, to suggest the child's gender by the shape of the belly or by the nature of the morning sickness, or even divine the future from tea leaves! This might make us less dismissive of beliefs of some cultures, such as that it is best to leave doors and windows open during labour, as it helps keep the cervix open, and, in others, that one should not step on ropes or cords while pregnant as doing so could give rise to a tangled umbilical cord! Here is a slightly more detailed example from another culture, the Madurese tribe in Indonesia,[58] a country which, in fact, has historically had high maternal mortality rates:

> The Madurese are typical of the many cultures where ritual is important, including complex ceremonies, food taboos, and a range of traditional practices, which in the case of the Madurese are very influenced by Islam. Some of the rituals here include both a fourth-month and a seventh-month pregnancy ceremony. They also have a tradition of pregnancy massage from the fourth month. This is thought to improve the baby's position, to reduce the mother's stiffness and fatigue, and facilitate an easier birth.

The fourth-month ritual takes place at a point where it is believed that the soul is 'blown into' the foetus. The ceremony includes inviting neighbours and reciting prayers, and at this time various good deeds are to be undertaken which are thought to ensure that the unborn baby will grow into a good moral person. Such acts include reading the Qur'ran and not killing animals. Stories abound, such as of the husband who cut off a frog's leg while his wife was pregnant, and the baby was born with a deformity of its legs.

They also have a ritual at seven months, which is more complex; this happens with a woman's first child, who is considered particularly important, a 'family successor'. The rituals include bathing rites that help purify the foetus, carried out with a traditional birth attendant, relatives, and religious leaders, and it involves pouring water mixed with flowers using a dipper made of coconut shells. There is also a ritual of preparing and carrying coconuts, one with Arabic letters on the outside and the other with Javanese letters, representing the complex cultural influences.

Again, the Madurese have a range of beliefs linked to pregnancy. For example, the pregnant woman is expected not to sit in a doorway, as doing so could lead to a more difficult birth while wrapping a towel around the mother's neck is thought to increase the risk of the baby being in danger from the umbilical cord.

The pregnant women are also encouraged to take various herbal and other foods and drink, including boiled turmeric and tamarind, which is said to refresh and clean the baby, moringa leaves to strengthen the baby, and coconut water to ease the birth.

Such rituals are deeply rooted in cultural and religious traditions and beliefs and reflect the ways in which the unborn baby is being brought into a community and its ancestral ways of being. This particular community has been able to link traditional practices and rites with newly introduced modern medicine, and this helps to increase safer births without losing its traditions. The support of the community, the rituals, the massage – these are exactly the kinds of things that help mothers-to-be feel safer and more held in their community and might well ease pain and labour.

When something big and potentially dangerous is about to happen, most of us will try to find a way to predict or even alter the future. For some, this includes rituals and prayer. In many cultures, this will include learning from one's ancestral past, and pregnancy is often assumed to be a time for linking to ancestors or spirits. In Maori culture the word *whānau* means both to give birth and also family, while *hapū* means both pregnant and clan, illustrating the significance of pregnancy and childbirth as a cultural phenomenon. According to the Ojibwe tribe of North America, the pregnant woman has 'one foot in the spirit world', so her dreams reveal messages about her unborn child. Dreams are also consulted for pregnancy divination among some tribes in Siberia. For Navajo people, pregnant women are seen as more spiritually potent, and there are strict protocols in place to protect mother and baby. Such linking of pregnancy to a spiritual life has a much smaller role in contemporary Western cultures.

Many decades ago, I visited the Dogon people of Mali. Here it is assumed that a woman becomes pregnant only with the permission of ancestor spirits called Nommo, who exist under the water. Ritual masks are used by men during sexual intercourse to summon the Nommo ancestors and request fertility. The child is, in many cultures, seen as a gift from ancestral spirits rather than arising solely from biological processes.

This might not be so different from some Western ways. Indeed, many Western parents name their children after ancestors. I, for example, was named after my great-grandfather, George, who was one of 17 children and needed courage to flee the pogroms in Russia before the revolution. He had to literally fight for his life to survive and then walk across Europe to the United Kingdom, while most of his siblings perished in Siberia. I still feel connected to him and his adventures.

Connecting to ancestors is important in many cultures, notably in Japan, where it is common to have shrines to ancestors in the home. In ancient Andean tribes, mother and foetus were symbolically wedded in a spiritual marriage ceremony, encouraging ancestral blessings. Vedic mantras chanted in India during pregnancy invoke divine protection of the growing baby.

Many of us feel relieved that these days we have the benefit of much modern medicine and information, but we might also feel that we are missing out on more traditional ways of connecting to a culture, its past, its beliefs, and the wider world.

CHAPTER 7

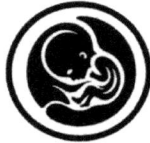

IS PARENTING SUPPOSED TO BE JUST ABOUT LOVE?

Parenting and pregnancy are by no means all joy, love, and ease. There are inevitably many difficulties and painful issues to face. For one, not all mothers want the babies they are carrying. I am aware that this is a somewhat taboo subject. As I have said, and it needs constantly reiterating, complex mixed feelings are part of life, of all relationships, including being a mother. We might not see this in most new-parent advice books nor on Instagram reels of super-mums, but becoming a parent is an emotional rollercoaster, one that might not be for everyone – or, at least, not at all times. Maternal instinct is not just there to be turned on, like water from a tap.

It is all too easy these days for parents to feel guilty, and to think that being a good or 'natural' (whatever that means) parent is all about being loving, caring, and compassionate. There can be something sentimental and guilt-inducing in how a lot of research, popular psychology, and newspaper columns describe parenting and children's development. Indeed, pregnant women often feel a big expectation that they should be thrilled and joyous about being pregnant, and mixed feelings can be hard for others to tolerate. As Jessica James told me:

> *You can feel very alone with your pregnancy. Everyone's excited on your behalf, but you might well have ambivalent feelings, alongside horrible physical symptoms, and you can feel awful and also quite isolated. So, connecting up with people is vital, at least after 12 weeks, when your pregnancy is more secure. Pregnant women benefit from belonging to a community with others, such as in antenatal groups, where it's possible to explore who you are and what you're going through, what your personal needs are, what your personal angle is on all of this.*

> *There ought to be some ambivalence. I worry about women who don't allow for more complex feelings. In my work, I always bring in the ordinariness of ambivalence. And, of course, everyone else often just thinks about the baby and not about you so much, especially later on. And pregnancy can be genuinely tumultuous for women. Of course, your life is going to change dramatically, and you can feel completely miserable because you are swollen, tired, and not feeling good in many ways. However happy you were to find you were pregnant and wanted to be pregnant, you can feel quite mixed about the actual experience and what it will be like as a mum with a baby.*

It is also worth remembering what research shows, that the needs, desires, and wishes of a child might not always coincide with a parent's wishes, and vice-versa, and that emotions that are often seen as more 'base', such as anger, resentment, or even rivalry, are all part of life, including parenting life. Let's be clear, nature is certainly not all about love and kindness; it can be ruthless and harsh, 'red in tooth and claw'. Like it or not, neither foetuses nor children are primed to live in a world of perfect mother–infant harmony. Conflict is engrained in all of animal nature, including human nature, as psychoanalysts,[59] and evolutionary psychologists such as Robert Trivers,[60] have long suggested. Parent and child share only half of each other's genes, at most, less when a woman carries an egg of a donor, or in recent cases of babies born with donor mitochondria in efforts to minimise specific health risks.

Science suggests that our genes drive much of our behaviour, and so different genes, especially if originating from different people, will have conflicting as well as common drivers and interests. Thus, perhaps surprising to some, conflict is inscribed at a cellular and genetic level. For example, it is in the interest of the foetus, not the mother, to transfer as many nutrients as possible across the placenta. The foetus's interests include increasing its own supply of sustenance, and one way of doing this is to send hormones into the mother's blood stream, which can raise maternal blood pressure, sometimes giving rise to symptoms ranging in seriousness from swollen calves to pre-eclampsia. Empathy is not, at this point, a part of the foetus's skill set! As Beth said:

> *I felt increasingly uncomfortable, and in particular, my legs and also feet had become swollen, and I felt heavy and bloated. You asked about bonding with the foetus, but at this stage I felt more resentment, even disconnection at times. I felt puffy, and unattractive, and tired. I really was not relishing the pregnancy.*

Swollen legs can in large part be due to the huge amount of extra blood needed to support a foetus that is looking after its own interests. From about five weeks, multiple messages pass from the embryo to the mother chemically. In fact, a pregnant mother's brain also undergoes rapid changes during pregnancy, and recent studies have shown[61], for example, changes in both grey and white matter, some of which last for several years postpartum, presumably helping ready a woman to become a mother. In fact, the embryo sends stem cells that colonise a mother's medulla, a central aspect of the nervous system; this has long-term effects as, in this process, lymphocytes, which are white blood cells – either B or T cells – become part of the mother's body and may remain so for decades. Some think there is a kind of organised cellular invasion from the foetus to the mother, with foetal stem cells colonizing the mother's body.

Perhaps invasion is too strong a term, but in recent years we have discovered a process called 'microchimerism', a term that comes from the Greek word 'chimera', which describes a creature made up of snippets of various animals. In microchimerism, there is trafficking of cells between genetically distinct individuals.[62] This often happens in pregnancy, via the placenta, and is thought to have a role both in some healing processes and also in some autoimmune issues. What this means, though, is that the DNA of another person can be inside us, and vice-versa. Microchimeric cells – including male ones which obviously did not start in the mother – have even been found in a mother's brain, all of which takes co-embodiment to another level, and challenges the myth of us being genuinely separate individuals.

After conception and during implantation, foetal cells that form what is known as the trophoblast invade and remodel the arteries in the mother's endometrium, so they are unable to constrict, these foetal cells literally stopping the mother withholding nutrients from the foetus. The human placenta has often been thought of as unusually 'invasive'. The foetus remodels the mother's arteries, so the mother cannot stop supplying it with nutrients without starving herself. We might describe this as the foetus establishing control of the territory to ensure its own growth. There is no sentimentality from the foetus here!

A mother's body develops its own response to foetal demands, so that a complex, mutually regulating tug-of-war type of process occurs. This, in fact, usually works out well. Sometimes, though, the balance is disturbed, such as when a pregnant woman contracts diabetes after the foetus's food demands lead to placental hormones increasing glucose too much. In such situations, the foetus could be thought of as self-interested. It releases hormones into the mother's circulation via the placenta to get the mother's body to act in a way that ensures that it, the foetus, receives the levels of glucose it needs. The mother's body generally counters this by producing more insulin, which normally (but not always) works out fine. It is when this goes too far that there can be a risk of gestational diabetes in the mother. The relationship between the foetus and maternal body is replete with such finely balanced tugs-of-war, each with a long evolutionary history.

The foetus also attempts to ensure increased blood flow to the placenta, which, in turn, pushes up the mother's blood pressure. Sometimes, but thankfully rarely, things get out of balance, and the mother's blood pressure drops; then the foetus, at risk of being starved of oxygen, ups the ante and releases toxins that constrict the mother's arteries, which increases blood pressure, and this can, in turn, cause horrible symptoms such as pre-eclampsia and even a risk of liver and kidney damage. Luckily these days doctors are well-versed in managing such eventualities.

Of course, the mother's body is also not driven only by love and compassion. Genes controlled by the mother limit foetal growth and ensure her own survival by making sure she is not depleted of all nutrients. So, rather than pregnancy being all about care and mutual support, we can also see a range of conflicts deep down at a cellular level, including between foetus and mother.

On top of this, the father's genome is also getting in on the act. Perhaps the best-documented of what look like conflicts takes place between the male and female genomes within the foetus. The biologist David Haig[63,64] was the first to study what he called genetic imprinting, which describes a process in which the same gene can express itself in different ways depending on which parent it is inherited from. In an extraordinary experiment with mice, either paternal or maternal genetic instructions were made inactive, thus on each occasion making only one parent's genome 'in charge' of a foetus. Male readers might not like this, but in foetuses where the mother's genome was driving the process, babies were born smaller but with larger brains, especially the parts to do with intelligence and complex emotional responses. On the other hand, those born by the rule of the father's genome were brawny and less clever! Even in pregnancy, conflicting, possibly selfish interests are engrained in our very genes and cell structure. It is easy to forget that we are not a unified being.

Using the word 'selfish' is perhaps not that helpful. After all, is it 'selfish' to even want a baby in the current world? There is even a philosophical school called *antinatalism* whose followers argue that it might have been better not to have been born.[65] Indeed, the decreasing birth rates in many parts of the world might attest to such a position. This was put graphically by one woman, Kes, who had had a cancer diagnosis, albeit a very hopeful one, and had always desperately wanted children, who said:

*It's hard to put your finger on why you want to have children,
but I have always known, since I was three years old. I have
worked with children and seen things that have been painful,
like children with nannies or in nurseries all day, and it made
me know how much I wanted children of my own. Just when I
was ready and we were going to try, I got a cancer diagnosis;
obviously that's a tough diagnosis. Thankfully, mine is
treatable. I have a loving partner and family but it's still scary
and I feel guilty, too; I want this so much, it's such a deep urge.
I can hear how selfish it sounds, but I cannot live with the idea
that cancer will take the one thing I have always wanted. I
know how difficult it is going to be.*

Is this selfish or just an extraordinary life force? It is far
from my right, or possibly anyone's, to judge, and if you want
to call this selfishness, it's the kind of selfishness that can make
someone into an extraordinary parent.

In terms of genes, more recent research[66] has taken this a
stage further and, using admittedly anthropomorphic
language, stated that genes controlled by the father are 'greedy'
and 'selfish' and will tend to manipulate maternal resources for
the benefit of the foetuses who, carrying the father's genes,
can then grow stronger. Although pregnancy is largely
cooperative, there is a big arena for potential conflict between
mother and baby, with imprinted genes and the placenta
playing key roles.[67]

Given the complexity of such processes, such as of
conflicting interests, it should be no surprise that most pregnant
mothers will experience some ambivalence. That is normal and
expectable and needs to be acknowledged and talked about,
rather than pushed underground and yield to cultural pressure to
be overly positive and ignore such mixed feelings.

Before closing the chapter, I need to acknowledge that sometimes the ambivalence can be stronger, and a baby might really not be wanted, which can have consequences down the line for both parties. Saying this is not intended to make any parents guilty at all – in fact, I would ban guilt if I could! I genuinely believe it helps to let people know that mixed feelings, and indeed negative feelings, are normal and common, and it behoves us to be as careful as we can to not judge anyone for their feelings. When we judge people's feelings, then those feelings can often go underground and be acted out unconsciously.

There is though interesting if painful data from studies of mothers who had, for example, asked for but were denied abortions. In Prague in the 1950s, abortion was made legal and more easily available, but some parents were not approved for such abortions. Researchers[68] followed some of these children whose mothers had been refused an abortion and compared them to a control group of children whose parents had never requested one. The less-wanted children did less well in school later and managed worse socially, had more health issues, and, as they got older, were more likely to have psychiatric issues. In addition, subjectively, they had less positive mindsets and experienced more anxiety. Perhaps worst of all, they fared less well in intimate relationships. Similar results were found in the large US Turnaway study,[69] which also showed that women who were able to have an abortion, many of whom were already mothers, fared much better later on in their lives as mothers, whereas children born to mothers who had wanted and been refused abortions had poorer outcomes.

On a similar note, one Canadian psychiatrist, Andrew Feldmar,[70] carried out interesting interviews with mothers of suicidal patients and found that many such patients had had mothers who had made unsuccessful attempts to abort their unborn children, and that, in fact, many had attempted suicide on the anniversary of the date when their mothers had tried to abort them. Others have reported similar results.[71] Such reports are mainly anecdotal, but it might be worth twisting this around a little: if, somehow, a pregnant mother's love can be transmitted to an unborn baby, might the same also be true of love's opposite?

As always, it is important to avoid judgement here and note that not everyone can be in a place to fall in love with their unborn baby. If this research is used at all, it should be as an argument for supporting mothers in whatever decisions they make and to provide emotional help in whatever way is needed, perhaps especially in providing spaces where their more difficult feelings, ones they might feel guilty about, can be heard and aired and accepted.

Many have argued that, in some circumstances, not seeing a pregnancy through might be a good option for a parent, if not for the unborn child. In hunter-gatherer societies, where conditions might support only one birth every four years, infants born too quickly were often left to die.[72] This, of course, was before abortions were available in the way they are now, at least in some places. It is worth remembering that, as cruel as it sounds, in our evolutionary history mothers often abandoned babies for a variety of reasons. We even have many biblical examples, such as Moses found in the bullrushes, or the putative founders of Rome, Romulus and Remus.

Sometimes such abandonment occurred because the father had been killed, or because circumstances had changed so that the mother could no longer enable the baby to thrive. In many hunter-gatherer communities, if a mother had twins, then breastfeeding might only be sufficient to keep one alive.

Timing is often crucial; a mother might abandon a child when circumstances are not propitious for childrearing yet might lovingly and devotedly care for another child born in more hopeful circumstances. Younger mothers living in poor areas are more likely to abandon offspring, perhaps believing that they will have other chances further down the line. During economic recessions, more babies tend to be abandoned.[73] The same points might be made about abortion, although I am aware that this is a controversial subject.

However, if a foetus is definitely going to go to term, there is genuinely much support we can offer to enhance the baby's chances of not only surviving but also thriving psychologically and physically. It is important that services and communities are alert to maternal ambivalence and work to ensure that the feelings of the pregnant woman are listened to and accepted, not judged.

There are many health professionals and services that can help, as well as friends and family and community groups. Interventions such as the Family Nurse Partnership in the United States and many other similar programmes offer support to pregnant women and girls who are living in challenging circumstances. The longer-term outcomes of those in such interventions have been fantastically hopeful, compared to those who did not have such support.[74] The results include better sleep, feeding, and emotional regulation after birth, and, in more serious 'at-risk' parents, less injury, hospitalisation, abuse, and developmental delay, as well as both better language and better cognitive functioning. Indeed, the research shows that right up until adolescence, there are gains for the offspring of those who were babies in the programme. We all benefit from support and feeling safe, and whether it is therapeutically informed care, a supportive community, or assistance with pressures such as poor housing and poverty, all such help makes a difference to later outcomes. But it is important to remember that some women will inevitably have mixed feelings about pregnancy, and that such feelings need to be taken seriously and, if possible, non-judgementally listened to and responded to compassionately.

I hope to have highlighted that some mixed feelings and ambivalence are part of most pregnancies and almost inevitable. Indeed, we have seen how much conflict is taking place at a cellular level, such as in how mother and foetus can have opposing interests. When you are feeling sick and your calves are swelling you should be forgiven for feeling some mixed feelings. After all, that little growing baby is looking after itself by, for example, getting as many nutrients from you as it can. Recent science has shown how much more than we might imagine is going on in this seemingly innocent process!

If there are any takeaways from this, it is that, sometimes at least, it is more than understandable to be irritated with a seemingly innocent being who might, in fact, at times have conflicting interests to yours! This is even more likely when a pregnant person is, for example, isolated, or has a trauma history or other psychological issues or is unable to emotionally care for even themselves. Obviously, we hope for loving, attuned, caring relationships, but this is not always possible. Aggression, anger, resentment, and rivalry are part of life. In fact, when they are denied and repressed, they can pop back up and do more harm than when they are owned up to, borne, and accepted. As psychotherapists know all too well, it is generally best not to deny or repress such negative feelings, because it is only the facing and processing of them that leads to them losing their power.

CHAPTER 8

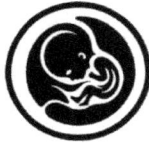

BEST ADVICE FOR THE FOETUS? CHOOSE YOUR PARENTS AND FOREBEARS CAREFULLY

It can seem unfair that one's parents' and grandparents' histories can affect not just us, but even our offspring and, indeed, possibly our offspring's offspring.

> *Joan had a very disturbed pregnancy in which neither her foetus nor she experienced much stillness. It was only during this pregnancy that she began to find out the stories about her own mother and grandmother. These included that her mother was born fleeing a war zone, where many of her family had perished. They nearly did not make it to safety because of her grandmother's pregnancy; indeed, her grandfather did not make it out. When my client was a foetus, her mother was gripped with terrible anxiety and reported expecting disaster throughout the pregnancy. Indeed, she witnessed many shocking events and*

had been subjected to unthinkable discrimination. Not surprisingly she was also very anxious throughout my client's childhood. The mother's understandably extreme levels of stress while pregnant and later clearly took their toll on my client's nervous system.

Yoga teacher Annabel Chown told me:

Before I got pregnant, I had already had a double mastectomy: I'd had breast cancer many years previously and subsequently discovered I carried a BRCA1 mutation, which put me at high risk of a new cancer. I knew the surgery would mean I wouldn't be able to breastfeed if I did become a mother. I worried that this would mean I was doing my child a disservice; that perhaps I shouldn't even become a mother if I couldn't give it my own milk? Equally, once I'd had the surgery, it was a huge relief to know that my risk of a new cancer had been reduced from around an 80% lifetime risk to less than 5%.

It is worth noting that while Annabel's situation was anxiety-provoking and difficult, it was nowhere near as extreme as in the first case. More importantly, her capacity to think about her own baby's needs and try to do the best for both of them is an important and positive prognostic sign, and you might not be surprised to learn that mother and baby, now a robust little boy, did really well.

In fact, a pregnant mother's capacity to think about her personal history, as well as being able to thoughtfully reflect on her own feelings, predicts her infant's behaviours a year or more after birth. In a fascinating experiment undertaken by Howard and Miriam Steele and Peter Fonagy,[75] pregnant first-time mothers were given a longish questionnaire called the Adult Attachment Interview (AAI). This is a tool that asks a range of questions about an adult's own early childhood. For example, it might ask them to think of five adjectives that describe their relationship with a parent or to remember experiences of being upset as a child and to whom, if anyone, they turned in such difficult moments. Another question was about what someone's memories are of early separations. What the interview really measures is an adult's capacity to make personal sense of their own emotional histories. What is especially being assessed is the adult's ability to reflect thoughtfully on their own experiences. The responses are coded into a few main categories. Some parents' responses are short and clipped, with little emotional understanding or nuance. Others are almost the opposite, with sentences that are very long and disjointed, very emotional, but with little coherence to the stories. The responses that predicted the most hopeful results, a secure attachment, were those in which the mothers were able to reflect honestly, thoughtfully, and reflectively while neither glossing over difficulties nor getting stuck in them.

What I find particularly interesting is that the important factor is not what happened to the mothers in their childhoods, but, rather, how they later, as adults reflected on and processed their childhood experiences. The quality (but not the content) of the mothers' interviews predicted with surprising accuracy the future attachment status of their as yet unborn child. In other words, it predicted the extent to which the children felt secure and confident, or anxious and clingy, or more cut-off or avoidant.

This suggests that the way we psychologically process our own emotional experiences and life histories is very linked to how we will likely also respond to other people's feelings, including any children we might have. It is the thoughtful, compassionate attention to emotions – our own and others' –

that leads to emotional and attachment security. A secure attachment style normally comes with more attunement to feelings, one's own and others', including one's child's.[76] This, of course, comes in large part from good support, whether a partner, friends, or wider family and community, or therapeutic support. Bad childhoods are not a life sentence. We can definitely 'earn' security by later having experiences in which our feelings can be heard and understood, such as in friendships, therapy, or support groups.

What the research suggests is that mothers who are more emotionally secure in attachment terms are also more able to be emotionally present to their infant's distress, to not be overwhelmed by it, and also better able to read their baby's emotional cues, than are less secure mothers, including those with more trauma-related attachment styles.[77] Our ability to form coherent narratives and self-reflective stories about our own lives can have a big influence on the emotional security of our as-yet-unborn children. A parent's emotional responsiveness also predicts how their unborn child will react to stressful situations at least a year after birth.

This is music to any therapist's ears, as most therapeutic work aims to help people become more accepting and aware of their emotional states. Of course, a baby, like any of us, benefits from being thoughtfully and caringly attended to. It is also likely that there will be continuity between a mother's states of mind during and after pregnancy, the family atmosphere, and the amount of stress and anger, or love and calm, before and after.

Such research certainly does not prove that the foetus's experience while in the womb is changed by a parent developing emotionally reflective capacities: such research is yet to be formally done. It does, though, still give us an incentive to trust in the importance of emotional support, especially during pregnancy, and also in the role of methods such as Raffai's prenatal bonding.

Foetal programming

We absolutely know that prenatal experiences have lasting influences in themselves, irrespective of what happens after birth. A well-known, if disturbing, example comes from the Second World War, where a cohort of Dutch mothers were literally starving and even resorted to eating tulips.[78] This state of starvation affected their foetuses, and this had long-term effects downstream. The foetuses grew into children and adults who had what are called 'thrifty' metabolisms, which in effect means that they used fewer calories and stored more fat, despite the food shortage no longer existing after their births.

This is an example of what is called 'foetal programming'. The pioneer of such research was David Barker,[79] and his work spawned large research programmes. The findings suggest that unborn babies can learn lessons to prepare for later life, which, in the case of the Second World War Dutch foetuses, would have been that food is scarce and needs conserving. Such a physiological strategy can be understood as a survival mechanism that takes root *in utero* – one based on the foetus adapting to its specific environment and predicting its future one. Apparently, as the title of one paper suggested,[80] *prescient human foetuses thrive*, and it seems that the foetus has great sensitivity to the signals it receives *in utero* and an ability to respond to these.[81]

In the case of the Dutch babies, such non-conscious biological predictions took root even though, in this case, it was not a useful strategy in their later lives in relatively affluent and food-abundant post-war Holland. It might feel bad enough that one puts on weight easily because of one's parents' unfortunate experiences long ago, but it gets worse. Many of these foetuses became adults who had a disproportionate number of other health and psychiatric issues. A similar effect of prenatal experiences was found in China. Mothers whose foetuses were affected by their malnutrition in the Great Leap Forward had offspring who later struggled at school[82] and were also more likely, for example, to suffer from cardiovascular disease as well as other health issues later in life.[83]

I have seen the effects of such experiences in my practice – for example:

> *A woman, whom I call Darsha, was seen in therapy for a number of years. She had made incredible changes in her life, but the last frontier was her relationship with food. She had always had problems with food, such as binge eating. Her life history had included being bullied, mistreated, and abused. She often talked about the psychological urge to eat and how it felt like a compulsion, but one she felt ashamed of. Indeed, she had been badly 'fat-shamed' by her parents and by others later in her life. We had assumed this had to do with her early experiences of neglect and abuse and had purely psychological precursors. However, she eventually discovered that when her mother had been pregnant with her as a very young woman, she had been very fashion-conscious, but also weight- and body-conscious, and in photographs looked almost anorexic. Darsha was born full-term but weighed only 4.5 pounds. This, shockingly, suggests she was near starving in utero. As a foetus she must have sensed that she lacked and badly needed nutrients and that there never was enough to sustain her, and as a preconscious unborn baby her biology would have led her to do*

her utmost to get what she could. I suspect that, rather than her being 'greedy', her biology was in part stuck in the world she had inhabited as a foetus, one of deprivation and an urgent need to, at all costs, get as much inside her body as she could.

This example seemed reminiscent to me of the Dutch babies whose mothers were starving in the Second World War.

It is also worth remembering that these effects can filter down to future generations too. Female foetuses, amazingly, already have about 4,000,000 eggs inside them, and these eggs and their physiology will also be affected by the prenatal environment of food deprivation, so that effects such as 'thrifty' metabolisms, and later healthy issues such as metabolic problems, might be seen for several generations. Life is cruel sometimes, but this is also a reason to take some of the pressure, blame, and self-blame off parents: we can do our best, but our destinies are partly out of our hands.

Such examples of foetal programming are extreme, but the principles of such research are hopefully relevant to all parents. The central tenet is that much of the foetus's physiology, its organs, nervous system, and brain, are being programmed during life as an embryo and foetus, as well as before conception. Prenatal experiences can give rise to physiological changes, some of which can be lasting.

Nutrition is, of course, very important, especially in the early months of pregnancy when cells are fast differentiating.[84] If there are not sufficient nutrients, then the foetus will learn to conserve energy, which can lead to a slower metabolism, which can, in turn, then be a predictor of later obesity. In thankfully very rare situations, the foetus might even end up relying on consuming its own body, such as its muscles, by processes such as gluconeogenesis. This is something that can also happen in adults who have insufficient calories to survive and who convert, for example, muscle into glucose. Very poor nutrition can influence gene expression, and, in some cases, we might see metabolic changes such as the production of hormones that inhibit growth and slow down metabolic rate. Again, this is rare in most countries in the West, but sadly less so for the global majority and, with rising inequality and poverty, is becoming less uncommon than we would hope in many so-called developed countries.

So, the somewhat glib headline is that we might do well to choose our parents, but possibly also our grandparents and even generations further back, very carefully. In fact, not only life before birth, but even a parent's and grandparent's lives before a baby is even conceived, can influence the as yet unconceived baby. For example, sperm can be affected by a father's history, which can impact how a range of genes gets expressed in the as-yet-unborn infant.[2] Similarly, a mother's germ cells, those that convey a parents' genes to the next generation, are affected by prolonged trauma exposure,[85] while in males, a clear effect has been found on foetuses and infants of both their father's stress and any excessive use of alcohol, as well as toxin exposure. In fact, a correlation has been found between maternal childhood trauma and the body size of an infant during the first year.[86] This makes sense intuitively and need not at all be anything to worry about, but it does mean that we might need to look further back in time for causative factors.

We still have a lot to learn about how long such effects last and when they 'wash out'. For example, in *Caenorhabditis elegans* (which, admittedly, is a worm!), stress effects have been found as far down the line as 50 generations![87]

While we might not find such clear and very long-term effects in humans or other mammals, new facts are being discovered all the time. A recent study showed that a mother's childhood experiences can be linked to DNA changes (methylation) in peripheral blood when she herself later becomes pregnant, these changes being seen in umbilical cord blood samples in newborns. This study[88] also found that such signs showed up in the quality of the intrauterine environment. Stress is a subject we come to in more detail in the next chapter. This is an example of some of the fascinating and fast-developing areas of recent research showing how a young female's early adverse childhood experiences (ACEs) can influence how their genes get expressed. This in turn will affect a range of physiological issues when and if that child eventually becomes pregnant herself.

Thankfully, the opposite is true, and what are called positive childhood experiences (PCEs) are increasingly being researched and have been shown to have a profoundly positive effect and, indeed, neutralise many negative effects of ACEs.[89]

The lessons from this chapter, and from much of the research in this guide, is that there is much we can and should do to support mothers and other parents and caregivers, and such support can do a massive amount to reduce worrying outcomes. The more good quality support there is, and the earlier it is given, the better.

CHAPTER 9

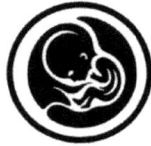

THINGS TO WORRY ABOUT?
STRESS AND WHAT WE PUT
INTO OUR BODIES

A foetus and mother cohabit, co-regulate, and share a world. The foetus is listening to music with the mother, moving with her as she moves, affected by her moods, thoughts, and feelings, by sounds heard *in utero*, and by a range of biochemical messages. Our fears, hopes, loving feelings, and anger all have biochemical correlates, and, while the foetus does not 'know' about our feelings, something of their effects get transmitted. We want our babies to do more than survive: we want them to thrive, and, in the case of the foetus, this means being physically well, healthily nourished, and, importantly, not overly stressed.

Stress

In this part of the chapter, I look at stress and talk about it in a way that, hopefully, does not lead to guilt or anxiety. Stress is something we need to recognise so we can do our best to avoid too much of it and give mothers and babies the best chance to flourish. I use the term 'stress' in the sense suggested by the founder of stress research, Hans Selye,[90] who saw it as a form of adaptation to challenges that is seen in the body as well as in the mind, with both psychological and physiological effects. Selye did not see stress as just bad, as it is also what can propel us towards growth and change if it is not too much for our systems to cope with.

When a mother becomes fearful, her heartbeat alters, often leading to reduced oxygen flow to the foetus or constricted arteries. In pregnancy, cortisol, probably the best-known hormone linked with stress, can cross the placenta, affecting foetal development. There are correlations between maternal and foetal cortisol levels, and some effects have been seen right up into adulthood.[91] One way of thinking about this is by using the metaphor suggested early on in this guide: that the brain and the body are constantly making predictions, at a physiological as well as a psychological level. Thus, the foetus is always making sense of its current environment and, seemingly, making (non-conscious) guesses about the future, almost like predicting the weather, and then responding at a physiological and possibly psychological level to these predictions. If it is likely to rain, I might prepare by getting an umbrella; if it is likely to be a scary world, I might prepare by readying myself for danger.

I want to add an important caveat here. When I talk about stress, I am meaning extremely high levels. Some stress is, in fact, good for the developing foetus in an otherwise stable pregnancy, and can even help the nervous system mature more quickly, and enhance cognitive and motor development.[92] No pregnant person should feel that they ought to be all bliss and calm, even if that were possible, which of course it most definitely is not. However, when there are very high levels of stress, which could be due, for example, to financial issues, domestic violence, racism, or extreme work pressures, then things might not work out as well. An enzyme in the placenta that would normally be able to stop cortisol crossing over to the foetus can, in fact, be blocked by a very stress-inducing environment.[93]

Extremely high – not average –levels of prenatal stress exposure have been linked to some birth complications, lower birth weight, and even prematurity.[94] David Barker was one of the first to show that low birth weight can often predict all kinds of diseases in adult life, such as coronary heart disease or Type 2 diabetes, and, indeed, early death, even when other factors such as genes or socioeconomic circumstances are screened out.[95,96] This should not be a cause of concern for most parents, as this is much more of a worry when there are insufficient nutrients, or when there are extremely – and I mean extremely – high levels of prenatal stress. It has, though, become increasingly clear that physiological matters like birth weight can be affected by stress or trauma – but this should never, of course, be thought of as a parent's fault. However, what we can do is screen as best we can and support anyone, including ourselves, who might be vulnerable and make sure that any of us can access the help that is needed.

When under stress a mother might sleep less, be more restless, absorb fewer nutrients and both mother and foetus will often thrive less well, which can affect brain volume[97] and motor development[98]. We might know this intuitively: when we are stressed and anxious, our arteries tend to contract and hence less oxygen and nutrients can pass through. High cortisol levels, it is hypothesised,[99] are among many psycho-biosocial factors that can lead to lesser growth in the foetus.

Indeed, unfair as this is, trauma in a pregnant mother's own childhood can predispose her to a range of worse outcomes.[100] Thus, blaming mothers (or mothers blaming themselves) is most definitely unhelpful and unwarranted. In such cases, we can and should make an extra effort to intervene and optimise the chances of a good outcome. Mothers with traumatic childhoods most certainly did not choose their early experiences, but if such parents can be helped, through therapy or good family or friendships or community support, then the risks can be minimised.

If we want to alter trajectories, then we owe it to future generations to face up to the potential risks and try to offer help where we can. I always try to be careful about discussing the effects of prenatal stress, as such research can all too easily trigger parental guilt or blame, which is most certainly not helpful. However, the more aware we are of potential risks, the more we can try to ensure that parents can get the support that they deserve.

Here are some of the more worrying facts (and this could be a moment to take a deep breath!). High-stress levels can alter the foetus's brain structure and sometimes be linked to later neurodevelopmental issues,[101] to mood and anxiety issues,[94] and to both cognitive and immune functioning.[102] Mechanisms such as cortisol crossing the placenta can lead to higher cortisol levels in an infant and altered postnatal stress systems.[103] Stress and anxiety in women during the Covid-19 pandemic, for example, has been linked to a range of postnatal issues such as infant negative emotionality.[104] However, research shows conclusively that such risks can be greatly reduced when sensitive attuned care is offered after birth.[105] Only if we do not offer such help before and/or after birth will we see the worst downstream effects.[106] It makes sense for future generations that we campaign and we try to ensure that at a national, local, and family level as much support as possible is available.

Of course, the impact of prenatal stress can be increased by living with equally stressed parents later, but stress during pregnancy has its own impact. Hence the need for investing in psychological and social support for pregnant mothers and their support systems, especially as interventions such as the Family Nurse Partnership, which includes visiting mothers pre- and postnatally, have been shown to deliver hopeful very long-term benefits.[107]

A particularly promising and well researched intervention has been developed by Catherine Monk and colleagues in Columbia University's Center for the transition to Parenthood. Their PREPP program (Practical Resources for Effective Postpartum Parenting), for example, screens pregnant mothers and foetuses for prenatal signs of potential worry, such as depression, poor nutrition, or psychiatric medication use, and offers support, both pre and postnatally; their findings are backed up by the use of rigorous scientific analysis, such as via fMRIs and careful blood sampling.[108] Given that maternal prenatal mind-mindedness, that is a parent's ability to be in touch with their child's minds and emotions, predicts better emotional regulation issues later in a child's life, this is another argument for prioritising compassionate and non-stigmatising prenatal family support.[109]

It is ongoing and repeated stress and trauma that have the most powerful impact. However, some stress derives from one-off rather than chronic experiences, and we also see effects if, for example, a mother experiences a sudden bereavement during pregnancy. Powerful effects have been seen when ordinarily well-functioning pregnant women are present at traumatising events such as 9/11[2] or terrifying hurricanes or ice storms.[110] Those involved in or in proximity to such disasters may end up with post-traumatic stress symptoms, and have children born with altered stress responses and cortisol levels. In such one-off stressors though, if reasonable support is available, the impact on the infant can be minimised and balanced by later positive influences.

However, generally it is social determinants, such as poverty, inequality, or degraded communities, linked to most of the worrying factors, whether drug or alcohol use or domestic violence,[99] that we should be most concerned about. These all take effect via a dysregulated nervous system, and at the risk of repeating myself, it is good emotional and social support, care and, dare I say, love, that are the best inoculation against the worst outcomes.

I have too often worked with cases where the causes were multiple and overdetermined, such as highly stressed mothers born into poverty and/or racism, who are the victims of violence or abuse and have little social support. Such a mother might be more likely to have a low-birth-weight baby and have birth complications, which can, in turn lead to difficulties in bonding. If one then adds the probability of intrusive medical attention, a decreased likelihood of breastfeeding, less attuned interaction, poor housing, and little support, then a baby's prognosis exponentially worsens. This is where professionals and services need to redouble efforts.

Social forces, biology, and psychology can interact powerfully. One perhaps surprising fact is that male foetuses tend to be more vulnerable and are less likely to even survive an extremely stressful prenatal environment.[111] Normally about 105 males are born for every 100 females, but when there is a great deal of stress, the number of boys born can reduce considerably. Such shifts in male foetal survival also happen at times of major social upheaval, such as war or economic downturns. In this and many respects, the male foetus is more fragile.

It is true that foetuses who are the result of unwanted pregnancies often fare worse, with more birth complications, poorer growth and less easy-going temperaments[26] than the very wanted babies who do better cognitively and have more secure attachments several months after birth.[112] It perhaps should not surprise us that accepted, loved, wanted, and planned babies fare better, but this should never be used as an excuse to condemn vulnerable women; they need help rather than criticism. Here again, we are seeing more arguments for building better relationships with babies from the time they are in the womb, which ultimately means building safer communities and support systems for the parents. We know that even when there is high prenatal stress, the downstream effects can be avoided when there is good social support in place after birth.[113]

Exactly the same caveats need to be made about the worries about what a pregnant woman might take into her own body. What is described here is probably well known and unsurprising; but I hope it is relevant to professionals and those with an academic interest, and that parents do not increase their stress or worry by reading it!

Substances

As well as stress, many substances, such as alcohol and both legal drugs such as anti-depressants[114] and antipsychotics[115] and illegal 'recreational' drugs,[116] can have some effect on the developing brain and nervous system. The first two trimesters are particularly vulnerable times. Clinicians who have worked with heroin-addicted newborns have described how their jerky desperate movements make excruciating viewing.[117] However, by far the most worrying recreational drug for the developing foetus is alcohol, very high levels of which can have a devastating effect on the vulnerable nervous system. Sadly, some children develop full-blown FAS (foetal alcohol syndrome),[118] with its classic set of dysmorphic facial features and its shocking effect on the brain and emotional and psychological capacities. Other infants escape the facial features but suffer from foetal alcohol spectrum disorder or FASD.[119] Their lives are often profoundly affected by this condition – some would even say blighted – as for such children, the brain areas involved in both memory and impulse control can be badly affected. These, though, are not issues that should worry most parents, as, while the jury remains out and academic debates continue, there is little evidence to suggest that there are any risks in having the odd glass of wine during pregnancy, even if some women prefer to avoid it. Indeed, many researchers bemoan what they see as the bigger risk of more mother-blaming and suggest that what poses far more risk to children is in fact a father's alcohol use, especially when it might come with worrying behaviours to mother or baby. In addition, high alcohol use shows itself in paternal sperm, which affects the foetus and baby.[120]

We might feel powerless when we realise things that we can do nothing about, many of which never would have been encountered previously in our evolutionary history. For example, air pollution has recently been linked to a whole range of later behavioural issues, as well as alteration in hormonal signalling, effects on brain areas such as the hippocampus, increased brain inflammation, and less of a vital substance, BDNF or brain-derived neurotrophic factor expression, which is a kind of fertiliser for the brain.[121]

Such findings, though, still leave many questions. For example, it is likely that those who experience more poverty or adversity also live in areas with higher levels of pollution. Do the most powerful effects arise from pollution, poverty, stress, or deprivation, or most likely, from a combination of these? Without doubt though pollutants can have powerful effects in their own right. Rather frighteningly, recent research showed that in a sample of the sperm of adult males, over 50% contained microplastics, which have been linked to reduced fertility.[122]

Women who became pregnant in the 1960s and 1970s, as Big Pharma was becoming more powerful, were often, unbelievably, advised to take sedatives, sleeping pills, and even benzodiazepines to improve their mood. They were often even encouraged to drink beer or wine, and shockingly, also to smoke, to help them to relax. Beer, in fact, was seen as a source of nutrients, such as selenium, potassium, and vitamin B; as a child, I well remember my neighbours swearing by the medicinal effects of Guinness for a pregnant woman. It was believed until not so long ago that the placenta would filter out anything of worry. No one knew about the dangers of toxoplasmosis from cat litter, for example. The placenta is incredible, but we should not overestimate its capacities. And we are learning all the time; I just discovered that babies whose mothers were using fentanyl have been born with a range of worrying features[123], such as microcephaly, unusual facial features and short stature, despite on the day of writing these words an UK NHS website suggesting it is safe to use[124].

Being exposed to smoking prenatally has also been shown to correlate with long-term effects, especially in terms of the later ability to self-regulate.[125] Adversity and factors such as inequality, racism, and their consequent stressors are clearly correlated with risks such as drug and alcohol use, pollution exposure, risk taking, and much more. The effect of maternal stress, anxiety, or depression on foetal development has been shown to hold up even when other factors such as biological inheritance, social class, diet, or smoking are screened out.[126] Once again there is a nature–nurture interplay. One study examined the effects of prenatal stress on mothers who were either pregnant with their own genetic child or one conceived via *in vitro* fertilisation (IVF) with a donor egg, lacking her genes.[127] In both cases, prenatal stress had a clear effect on later behavioural problems, but this was slightly greater in a child conceived using the mother's eggs. In other words, some, but not all, later behaviour was influenced by genetic inheritance, with both genes and environment playing a role.

Just because stress or maternal alcohol or drug use can lead to low birth weight and other issues, we should on no account focus on, nor ever blame, stressed mothers for the physical and emotional health of their offspring. This research takes us far beyond the responsibilities of the individual parent. Stress, anxiety, or substance misuse do not occur by chance or in a vacuum. They increase for those socially and economically marginalised, and particularly for those who are poor in an unequal society,[128] or are the victims of racism[129] or of domestic violence or abuse. We might think of these physiological sequelae as ways in which social forces, inequality, poverty, and the like are expressed in the bodies of mother and foetus.

We could argue that maternal substance abuse and stress levels are both caused by, and a signifier of, social, political, economic, and cultural issues. If responsibility lies anywhere, it is with society, rather than with individual parents. We should perhaps take courage from research that has shown that incredibly, but also hopefully, when a US State invests in programs to alleviate poverty and economic hardship, we actually see benefits in terms of the brain development as well as mental health of the offspring living in the communities that are given financial help.[130] Such issues are always about more than parenting, but nonetheless we can still do our best to ensure that parents can help their offspring to have the best chance, including in prenatal life.

CHAPTER 10

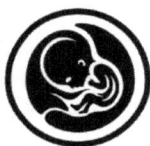

BIRTH

Now it's time to think about birth. As pregnancy nears its end, it makes sense that there are varying degrees of both dread and eager anticipation of the birthing process, as well as a longing to meet the baby. As Valerie, whose birth is described later in this chapter, said:

> As time went on, I could feel myself becoming impatient to know my baby more fully. I longed for the birth and the possibility of meeting this new being who I felt so attached to and yet was still so hidden.

This was poetically echoed by my colleague Emily:

> If only the door didn't have to open at some point – that was a scary and unthinkable venture and at first took quite some speaking to women who had been there and knew. I found myself reaching for grounding and earth and a steady reminder of the wisdom of a woman's body.

Nature helped me out eventually as I began to feel it was impossible to move my gigantic form any longer and the inevitability of exit became firmly planted in my mind.

I had long by now become public property: somehow one's protruding stomach is license for everyone to give you 'advice' on what you should be doing – e.g., not cycling, even if it is much easier than walking! I knew I could make some fairly sensible decisions based on what I knew was going on in my body not theirs, and how to safely conduct myself and trust my feelings.

While most of this guide focuses on prenatal life, I here look at some important aspects of the birth process, especially those linked with psychological and emotional issues.

Active birth teacher and group psychoanalyst Jessica James helpfully explains how, in fact,

… the whole experience of pregnancy is preparation for the experience of birth. which is, in turn, preparation for parenthood. There are all the kinds of things that happen to your body, like the unpredictability, the attention your body needs, emotions being all over the place, and the unsettledness. The birth is the most extreme part of this because, for a start, you don't know when you're going to go into labour. You don't know when it's going to happen, and even when it does start, you don't know how long it's going to be. It might be 3 hours, 30 hours, or even longer. No one knows how the birth is going to go, even when you're in it. The most experienced midwife can't predict that. It's something about bearing the unknown and managing the unpredictability. And then there's the loss of control, of your bodily functions. There's water and liquid, even faeces, all over the place, and you're probably making lots of animal-like noises. And when you've got the baby, it's the same unpredictability, about sleep, feeding, illnesses, routines, moods,

everything. When you put down a newborn baby, sometimes it sleeps for three minutes, at another it's three hours!

I've learned over the years that it's not the type of birth you have that leaves you traumatised, it's the way it was handled. What counts is the extent to which you understood what went on and the amount of control you had over how it went, but also how informed you are. You might unexpectedly need to have a caesarean but feel absolutely fine about it because you understood why it was needed and you were involved in the decisions. What's really traumatic is when something's done to you and you feel completely out of control, and you don't really understand why. Some women have what sounds like the most horrendous birth in terms of the actual facts of it but feel ok and are able to emerge positively. It's most important that a woman feels 'I did my best', 'I felt looked after'. It can be a big letdown to be told that if you do what I tell you, then it's all going to be all right, as can happen in some approaches to birth preparation, and then it doesn't happen in that way.

James' point here is crucial. For example, many mothers have felt, or even have been made to feel, that their birth was somehow inferior if it was via caesarean section. However, as some stories here attest, often it is the best option, and, if done well, these days in the form of what is often called a 'gentle C-section' or a 'family-centred caesarean birth', then the experience can be quite beautiful and rewarding.[131]

Birth is more hazardous and painful for humans than for most species. The traditional view is that of the obstetric dilemma, which suggests that this is due to a combination of the relatively large size of our brains and the small pelvises that developed several million years ago when our forebears became bipeds.[132] It is certainly true that human infants are born relatively immature but with a brain large enough to be extraordinarily flexible, enabling us to adapt to almost any culture and environment. It might well be that our large brains have, literally, painful costs. The obstetric dilemma evolutionary view has, however, recently been critiqued by Holly Dunsworth,[133] who suggests that there is not enough evidence for this theory and there are other possible explanations, such as metabolic ones. More worryingly, she suggests that this theory can be used to justify all kinds of interventions, such as inductions and caesarean sections, when they might not be necessary. This too often happens instead of providing birthing environments in which women are encouraged to trust their senses and be allowed to be in control of the process as much as possible.

The experience of birth nearly always leaves a profound psychic mark on women. I am always surprised when I teach about child development, that of all the many subjects on the syllabus, birth evokes the strongest feelings and the most personal and powerful memories. When doing interviews for this book, someone told me how, when they were pregnant, they couldn't seem to stop other women coming up to them, completely unsolicited, with their birth stories, many of which were frankly traumatic, and this only made them feel more stress. One person told me how an 84-year-old whose great-niece was pregnant, insisted on sharing her traumatic birth stories from sixty years ago. The experience seemed as alive now as it was all those decades ago, but this storytelling was not appreciated by the niece! I have heard this often enough to realise that in fact women need protection from other women who might need to offload their stories and that being a good listener might come with a price, especially to one's own stress levels.

How a birth pans out varies hugely, of course, from person to person, and also across cultures and historical periods. Something seen as 'natural' in one era or culture might seem very alien in another. Until recently, the use of stirrups for birthing was *de rigueur* in Western hospitals, and across the Western world in recent decades caesarean section has been on the increase. Many women today want what are called 'natural' births, nowadays often with fathers present. In Holland, home births are common and, indeed, encouraged by the government, assisted by what they call a *kraamverzorgster,* who specialises in such care. Similarly, in Sweden prenatal and postnatal care is free, and mothers can choose between giving birth at home or in hospital and can also access alternative pain relief options such as acupuncture. In fact, acupuncture has traditionally been and still is often used in China for pain relief.[134]

Although the attendance of fathers at births is now common in many Western societies, until recently in most societies, males attending births was unusual. In colonial North America, for example, husbands were not allowed to witness a birth. In pre-modern Europe and much of the Middle East, this has also been the case. However, this modern trend is not unique. In many Native American groups, such as the Navajo and Hopi, men participate in a birth ceremony, and this is seen as a sacred communal act. There is no one 'natural' universal way to approach birth, although in most cultures it is the presence of supportive older females that is more usual.

Some ask if it is even right for fathers to attend births? Most parents I spoke to who were in heterosexual relationships wouldn't have had it any other way. Most women were very grateful for a father's presence, and most fathers feel honoured, and many see it as a life-defining experience. However, some have worried that there can be pressure on men, when some can be emotionally ill-equipped. As Nikita Akilapa told me:

> *I have witnessed some wonderful birth partners who were engaged and invested and totally present mentally, emotionally, and energetically. These are the birth partners who positively influence birth. I have also encountered some who are only there physically because they've been asked to be there, or because they know that they really should be. But if they're not fully present, for whatever reason, then it can have a detrimental effect. The person who is trying to give birth, whose maternal caring instincts are in overdrive, will likely be extending her care to worrying about you, when it's actually she who needs looking after. And if she doesn't feel held and cared for, she may also not feel safe, which can interfere with the process of birth.*

Birth expert Michel Odent has also suggested[135] that a father's presence can sometimes be detrimental, increasing a mother's anxiety and also affecting the father's mental health. That, thankfully, has not been my experience, nor that of most of my peers, and most partners I spoke to felt very grateful for the support of their partner, most often a father. In fact, sometimes there is literally no choice. One good friend of mine ended up catching the baby as the midwife was delayed, and this is not that uncommon. Nikita gave me another example:

> *I supported a couple who gave birth to their second baby at home. It was so quick; the baby was born before either myself or the midwife arrived. During our antenatal sessions, we had discussed whether or not Dad might like to catch the baby. He had said that he wasn't keen on that at all, because he's a bit squeamish. His actual words were, 'I don't want to be at the*

*business end!' But on the day of the birth, given no other option
but to catch his baby, he rose to the challenge beautifully. When
he opened the door to me, he was elated and so proud of himself.
Mum felt incredibly safe and supported and felt that this had
been a unifying bonding experience. Interestingly, they told me
that this time around, the dad is so much more involved in the
postpartum nurturing.*

There are many variants of what are called natural – or,
sometimes, 'physiological' – births, but what they generally
have in common is the aim of giving the woman more control
over the birth process. In the Western world birth has become
highly medicalised, and in some countries, the risk of legal
action can mean that doctors can be very cautious. The
advantages of this are, obviously, that for mothers and infants,
mortality rates are much lower, but those in the natural birth
movement argue that in such medicalisation something has
been lost as well as gained.

Natural birthing ideas have been much influenced by
practices of more traditional cultures. For example, in many
birthing classes, women are taught to give birth in the
squatting position, just like, for example, the Himba of
Namibia, who give birth squatting in a hut accompanied by
female relatives. Indeed, in many Māori societies births took
place in sacred womb-like shelters, called *whare kōhanga* and
during birth, mothers would usually squat and hold on to
handposts; similarly many indigenous Australian women will
also walk during labour and squat in the later stages. There are
multiple cultural variations on how to give birth: the practice
in ancient Egypt was for the woman to give birth on a special
birthing stool surrounded by female relatives and friends;
possibly unusually, the Bariba women in Benin are expected

to be strong in the face of pain, in fact, gain respect and social kudos from solitary birthing.[136]

Water births have become more sought after in Western cultures, and they too have a long tradition: the Shipibo people of the Amazon, for example, use a steam bath called a *temazcal* to induce labour, while in Hawaii many births have traditionally taken place via under-water delivery, designed to make the birth process smoother. While the Western natural birthing movements have learnt much from such cultures, it is probably true to say that in the West birth, and indeed pregnancy, are viewed primarily as biological and medical processes, whereas in most indigenous communities it is a more spiritually imbued process and a way in which ancestral traditions are passed on.

We do not know if there is any medicinal benefit in the Zuni Native American tradition of rubbing cornmeal on the belly to bless the child. Certainly, few readers would hold much faith in medieval European rituals such as laying a sword under the bed to cut pain or putting a key on the belly to unlock the womb. However, we can be pretty sure that in such ritual acts the sense of community, of being held by family and tradition, and of feeling cared for were almost definitely easing pain and making for a smoother birth process. In fact, though, some women I spoke to had clearly been able to make the link between their current births and their ancestral history; take Merrilyn:

> *My first pregnancy happened shortly before the days when a simple scan would reveal the sex of your child, but it was no surprise to me that our baby was a girl. Throughout my pregnancy, I had been certain that the child within me would be a little girl with brown eyes. I could imagine no other, I felt very close to my baby long before she was born. She was conceived in*

a special area of Pembrokeshire in October 1976. I am not sure I told her that: too much information, people would say! However, she was most definitely imbued with the spirit of Pembrokeshire throughout her life, probably from that day. The earth, rocks, and sea from which many generations of her ancestors had sprung were, for her, tangible, real, alive.

Merrilyn's awareness and respect for her cultural and natural history is perhaps not very common in the contemporary world. Every culture has its own way of doing things, and we should be prepared to admit the possibility that what we assume to be the right way might not be how everyone else sees it and that practices that might seem odd in one culture can seem normal in another, and vice-versa. What we think of as cutting-edge knowledge today can tomorrow seem a quaint superstition, and views based in different cultural worldviews can be a challenge to our beliefs or biases.

Some birthing stories

Here is Anne's account of a second pregnancy and birth, which went very smoothly, after she had learnt painful lessons in a difficult first birth:

I knew that I wanted to have another baby. I felt like I'd missed something by having two babies at once and wanted to have an opportunity to look after just one baby. I had a strong premonition that this time we would have a boy, and I felt like it would be ok. I'd had some more therapy by then! I fell pregnant straight away, and this pregnancy was much more straightforward.

I felt happy and bonded from early on, and I felt tiny flutters of movement as early as the end of the first trimester. I had expected that to be the case, and I didn't feel disturbed. There was a degree of stress towards the end of the pregnancy, caused by naively doing building work, and looking after my toddler twins of course made it more tiring, but I was able to read books about positive birth experiences and do hypno-birthing meditations and yoga. I went into labour two weeks early. In a rather comical fashion, I went into extreme nesting mode, and my kind friends from next door joined me in donning rubber gloves and trying to clean up the building dust and prepare the house. By 11 pm the contractions were less than four minutes apart. I knocked on the taped-up kitchen door, where my husband was trying to fit a sink, and his precise words were, 'not now!' Apparently, he was trying to do the silicone seal at the time! I insisted, and we got on our way to the hospital.

In less than two hours, he had arrived safely, a big chunk of a baby at almost 10 pounds. It was an un-medicated birth, I felt so well prepared by what I had read and able to deliver in the way that felt natural to me. We had all the skin-to-skin we liked this time, and he just got on with feeding with no problems, and we went home the next morning. Despite the ongoing chaos in the house, this time I felt empowered by the birth, and was in a serene mental space. I loved holding and feeding my son, especially in the evenings, when the girls were in bed.

I often used a sling with him and didn't worry about where he napped, so if it was easiest to hold him when he napped, that's what we did. There was none of that second-guessing my own decisions which had taken up so much energy when becoming parents for the first time. The ease of this pregnancy and birth were, I think, linked to how things went afterwards. He was a contented baby, and easy to look after. During that first year we used to joke that you could sometimes forget he was there, he *would just nap in the Moses basket while noisy life went on around him. He is now 6 and thriving.*

In Anne's case, much was clearly learnt from the natural birth movements and from her own previous experiences, as well perhaps as from something similar to that espoused in Raffai's prenatal bonding methods.

As early as the 1970s Klaus and Kennel piloted schemes in which supportive women stayed with the mother throughout the birth, and the result was quicker births and fewer complications.[137] In one study, 240 first-time mothers were randomly assigned either to a group who were given a 'doula', or to a control group whose births were managed 'as normal'. The supported mothers had fewer caesarean sections, the babies had less meconium staining, which is a typical sign of a distressed foetus, and were less likely to be hospitalised in the postnatal months. Indeed, research suggests that continuous midwife care shortens labour and reduces birth complications.[138] Generally supportive attachment histories and caring current relationships make the birth process go much more smoothly.[139] The importance of psychological support can never be underestimated, and it begins very early.

The release of the much-talked-about neurotransmitter, oxytocin, is probably central. We release oxytocin when we bond with someone, feel good, make love, and during labour as well as in breastfeeding. It enhances immune responses and protects against physical (and social) pain; we produce greater doses when feeling supported and cared for. Many other chemicals are also naturally released, such as adrenaline and noradrenalin, and the possibly under-rated beta-endorphins, all of which reduce pain and make the birth process more manageable.

The Active Birth Movement has had a powerful influence, empowering women to take more control of the birth process,[140] not least in ensuring that women have the best support and information. In recent years we have seen the rise of many popular methods for facilitating easier and less painful births, perhaps especially hypnobirthing and mindful birthing. Hypnobirthing has become increasingly popular, and I am sure is familiar to many readers. It uses methods such as breathing techniques, positive imagery, and language, as well as visualisations to work against the idea that birth has to be painful and difficult.[141]

Maria told me:

> I took an online yoga class for pregnancy and birth with a friend. It included a mother's support group on What's App. I learned different breathing techniques, support for birth, and also connected to my baby through somatic sounds. In one of the meditations, we connected my heart with the foetus's through a green-golden line.
>
> I also took a prenatal class with my husband, so that he would know what to do. I had a very easy pregnancy, the worst of it being a few cramps and slight breathing problems. In the pregnancy yoga class, we told each other how we were in every session, and I learned that I was very lucky that I felt so well during the whole pregnancy, not even having any nausea.
>
> The only fear I had was of not having a natural birth and ending up with a caesarean which (spoiler!) I did in the end, despite doing lots of hypnobirthing and positive thinking. The classes helped me stay calm during pregnancy and I was always confident. I never thought that something would go wrong.

There are many studies, such as of hypnobirthing, and also of mindful birthing, initial research about which looks very promising. In mindful birthing the idea is not so much to change a birthgiver's core experiences as to be more compassionately present to the feelings and sensations that are actually there, with the idea that being self-compassionately present in itself changes the experience. For example, the anticipation of the pain of the next contraction might mean that mothers tense up, and in fact such tensing increases pain when the next contraction does come, which can stop a woman from making the best use of the naturally occurring soothing opioids between contractions[142] – opioids that are probably more powerful than expensive street drugs! It does seem from research overviews that no one intervention is better than any other; there are studies looking at a range of interventions that look promising, and in fact all helped to reduce the fear of childbirth.[143]

This is not to say that the pain is not nearly always awful and can sometimes feel too much to bear. As Emily told me:

> *A kindly midwife, who had given birth to five of her own, reminded me, 'when you feel like you are going to die, the pain then eases.' It was true! It was completely true! It just peaks, and then it is down the other side again. With that vital piece of information – which, you would have thought, I could have observed for myself, except I was in truth starting to freak out – meant the world of difference. It no longer felt like pain really, just the most intense and weird tunnel someone had put me through in which I had no control other than to focus and to keep accepting the daunting prospect of opening – or is it exiting or letting go or dying, or admitting I have no clue (and by the way does anyone else in the room?). But this was something that requires a lot of trust.'*

A take-home message must be that women who experience skilled and compassionate support during pregnancy are far more likely to have an easier birth. The caveat is that things do not always work out well, often due to sheer bad luck. Of course, a pain-free birth or one with minimal interventions is the ideal, but there is a danger that this becomes a standard against which women can judge and blame themselves and even consider themselves a failure. That is not helpful. As Annabel Chown, my friend and yoga teacher, told me:

> *I had hoped for a natural birth, and dreamed, like many, of the birthing pool, the beautiful playlist, essential oils, and an experience that was intense but beautiful. I read books on hypnobirthing, I visualised my baby coming out naturally and easefully into the world. That said, I wasn't going to strive for a natural birth at any price. I'd waited a long time to have a baby, and the most important thing was he arrived safely.*

> *Because I was over 40, the doctors recommended I didn't go over my due date, which can apparently increase the risk to the baby. They suggested an induction if labour hadn't started by then. But having heard of so many friends, especially those over forty, go through inductions that ended up in emergency C-sections, I decided that if my son hadn't appeared by my due date, I'd prefer the calm of a planned C-section.*

> *This was booked for the day after my due date. And even when I woke up that morning, I hoped labour would kick in naturally, and the surgery, booked for that afternoon, wouldn't need to happen. Once it got to noon, I realised this was a dream I'd have to let go of, and I cried a bit.*

> *While I wouldn't have chosen a C-section, in the end it had its own beauty: the knowing, as I was prepped for it, that within the next hour I'd meet my son. The operating theatre with so many people attending to us, the professionals caring that this all went well. The song we'd had for our first dance at the*

wedding (a Coldplay one) coming on just as my son was taken out of my body. And his safe and calm arrival onto my chest.

While it is true that many of these and other interventions can give women and babies the best chance of coming through the birth process as well as possible, none are foolproof. There can be a lot of pressure in some circles to give birth 'naturally', and sometimes this does not feel right and is rightly resisted. Debbie had had a traumatic first birth. She told me that next time:

When I was about to have my second child, I insisted on a C-section, as I was not going to have a repeat performance. I went into labour and had my requested C-section. The birth was calm, I recovered quickly, and I bonded instantly with my second daughter. No post-natal depression. I did, however, get a lot of criticism from both my family and others for making this decision and not 'allowing' my baby a natural birth. I have wondered about this element of control or lack thereof as I've spoken to other mums about their birth process. I wonder to what extent the experience of the birth and the mother's feelings of being heard and held and allowed to make decisions that affect her go on to then affect her relationship with her infant.

Support is so important

One of the time-honoured ways of providing support that has proven to be effective is the use of doulas and other forms of supportive birthing partners. Such birthing support has been shown[144] to have many hopeful outcomes, including a reduction in premature births, as well as in caesarean sections, less use of pain management including epidurals, and shorter labour times. Such outcomes seem to be associated with a reduction in stress and anxiety, the support in itself giving rise to the release of pain-reducing neurochemicals such as oxytocin and beta endorphins. The presence of doulas also improves outcomes after birth, including better sleep and more success in breastfeeding. One hopeful finding is that women from lower socioeconomic backgrounds, who have tended to have worse outcomes, in fact closed this gap significantly when they had doula support. Unfortunately, doula-type support is beyond the means of many women who need it most.

Emily's example will speak to many women:

> *At the moment of labour, I found myself wanting people to take care of my body and me and my baby's progress as the contractions started in earnest. I realised that I had to kind of die to give birth, by which I mean, surrender, there is absolutely no other way to survive those major contractions, particularly those that happen at the end. They wholeheartedly feel like they will surely take you out for no human could withstand the power that was in them. Tremendous power, pain, yes, but power, and totally outside my control, my body and not my body. That is an experience I never had before or since.*
>
> *And yet both me and my precious parcel, my loved one with whom a whole relationship had been firmly established, were on the other side of these contractions, each one in their compartment. Each one having to accept that this is it, separation and unknown futures and spaces are coming.*

Psychological factors such as stress have an impact on the quality of a birth as well as a pregnancy. This is why, as previously said, it is incumbent upon us, as professionals, parents, family, friends, and partners, to ensure that there is as much support as possible, remembering how good social connection reduces stress and makes us feel safe. Pregnant mothers with little support, or with histories of adversity, often release less oxytocin but higher levels of cortisol and can be at more risk of earlier and more difficult births as well as of postnatal depression.[145] The presence of a supportive, empathic, and experienced person nearly always helps and can ease and speed births and reduce the risks of complications.[146,147]

Women who have more adverse childhood experiences (ACEs) are more likely to have more social and psychological issues, and these can impact on the birth process as well as later bonding. It seems unfair that one set of bad experiences can increase the likelihood of later ones at this crucial time. However, I believe this is all the more reason not to ignore factors such as ACEs but, rather, to try to ensure that we screen or look out for risk factors and then offer extra help to those who might need it. This can make a big difference.

Shockingly, preterm birth is far higher in black women – something that research has struggled to explain in a satisfactory way. Recent studies have looked at a wide range of factors, including diet, microbiota, hypertension, depression, socio-economic conditions, exposure to pollutants, but taking such a huge array of factors into account, in the end it is looking most likely that racism plays the biggest role at many levels, including in exacerbating stress, giving rise to a lifetime of health issues as well as disparities in the quality of actual care received from medical staff.[148] The other effects, such as health differences, poverty, exposure to pollutants, inflammatory issues, might also be explained as downstream of the experience of racism.

The take-home message must be that all women need respect, support, care, and for their specific needs to be taken seriously, and – less scientific perhaps but most importantly – they need love and compassionate support. Those who are more marginalised face a much bigger challenge to receive the help they need so that they can give their unborn babies the best chance of being healthy, happy, and thriving. It is women like Arya who need more of our and society's support, and all too frequently get the opposite:

> *As a care-experienced adult and person of colour, my experience of giving birth was doubly challenging. My first-born was, unexpectedly, 6 weeks early, and my early life experience, while helping me to disassociate and go with whatever was going to happen, meant I did not have the confidence to protest or demand the best options. Arriving at the hospital 20 mins after my waters broke and contractions two minutes apart, I was told to stay in the waiting area. I was in agony and was not seen for 30 mins before I begged my husband to speak to someone.*

> *I was practically on all fours in front of other couples, and I was told that I could not be in labour. When I was eventually seen, the midwife said 'shit, she's 9 centimetres dilated' and took me to a room where I was put on my back with a heart monitor for my baby's heart. I had no pain relief at all and was not offered any. I constantly said to the midwife that being on my back was not helping and that my body was naturally pushing me to be on all fours, all of which was ignored.*

Arya's experience is shocking but all too common, especially for women of colour. Some women, often those with more privilege, are better able to ask for that help and know what they want. A beautiful example came to me from Merrilyn. You might remember Merrilyn, whose first baby, Megan, was born imbued with feelings for the Pembrokeshire countryside?

> *Megan in time became a mother herself, as well as an equine veterinary surgeon, a poet, musician, a wife, a mother, poet, and*

a passionate horsewoman. Her mother, Merrilyn, described her[49] as 'gifted, headstrong, compassionate, tempestuous, beautiful, and wise'. Megan was totally opposed to the idea that birth was a medical procedure and adamant that her baby would be born at home. She had been present at numerous animal births and saw the arrival of new life as a totally natural event. Her son was delivered by an independent midwife, Virginia, who became a friend. She and Megan were two of a kind. Strong women. They understood each other. When Virginia asked Megan what she wanted from her midwifery care, Megan said that she had no intention of getting on a 'conveyor belt of care' and told Virginia: 'I want to be in charge! My body, my pregnancy, my labour, my baby. I want to feel I have the best information available in order to form my own judgements and make my own decisions about my care and that those choices will be supported. I do not want my needs subjected to someone else's perceived notion of what is best for the baby.' Megan had told Virginia that the birth was going to be like a party. I remembered thinking that it could all change on the actual day of the birth, because birth can be tough, but in the event it really was like a party. 'No drama, no fuss, and on a cold January day Megan birthed a beautiful, healthy, strong son at home on the farm she loved with the husband she loved, exactly like she had predicted and just like the strong, confident woman I know'.

In fact, such births seemed to run in Merrilyn's family. She wrote:

All three of my grandchildren were born at home and delivered by the same midwife, Virginia. Megan felt so strongly that birth was a natural event that she introduced her midwife to her sister so that she too could experience a good home birth - which is what happened. There were no problems or complications. I too was born at home because, in the years after the war, there was not enough space in hospitals. In fact, giving birth at home used to be the norm but these days we have medicalised it and hospitalised it. The key difference I would say is that the mother feels relaxed and comfortable at home, as long as she knows she is in the hands of a competent midwife, and this is key to a 'good birth'.

So, there are good, moving stories, and sometimes, but very rarely, birth is unexpectedly and enviably easy, as recounted by Bianca, a daughter of a friend:

I had my baby at 28 years old, and everyone warned me how painful it would be. In the labour ward the doctors kept coming up to me to check if I was all right, and they were astonished that although I was having contractions very close together, I felt almost nothing, no real pain, hardly any discomfort. The doctors then came over to monitor me with a machine. One said, 'look at the screen, see the waves of your contraction? and when a big wave came they asked, 'what can you feel?' I could only give the same answer, 'I feel almost nothing!' In fact, I was so relaxed they had to tell me, in fact shout at me, to push, one even threatened me with induction. But in fact even the final part of the process was easy and pain-free, so much so that I barely knew when my lovely son, Adam, had been born.

Now, this is very unusual, something I have only ever seen watching videos of the enviably easy births of non-human primates! Perhaps women should not get their hopes up!

Here is a more hopeful experience from Valerie, where things went pretty well.

It is rare, I know, but it all started exactly on my due date, which was a relief, as being an elder mother, nearly 40, I was worried about the pressure from the medical team. My waters broke, a bit like a sudden gush from nowhere, and then we waited and measured the timing of contractions. So, it was going to really happen! It had started! I, helped by my partner, began to do the breathing exercises, and spontaneously, on bad contractions, we did some (it might sound weird) chanting; the long outbreaths really helped. This was mid-afternoon.

By later in the evening the contractions were getting more frequent and painful. My lovely neighbour, Jen, took us to the hospital, equipped with music, clothes, and brandy for my partner(!). All was smooth getting into the hospital, but, although we had planned to have the birthing centre with a pool, it was a bank holiday and it was closed, which was disappointing but not terrible. We had our own room, and labour was getting established, and my lovely friend in fact stayed, although this was not planned.

My husband was by my side the whole time, holding my hand, and we were breathing together, and I just got into a zone. Jen was a huge help, I was screaming at times, and she would massage my back and hum and sing, and I felt very loved, although I was not very present to anything outside my body. We were offered gas and air, but somehow, I did without and managed by staying present and focused. I could certainly tell when the transition started.

There was a change of staff, which felt a bit unsafe, but in fact the new midwife was lovely, although she just popped in and out. It was really my husband and Jen, and I felt them there the whole time. They breathed and chanted with me, and we breathed more and more deeply. At times I lost it and came into the pain but could re-establish myself in that zone. Before the changeover there was pressure to start pushing. I knew I was not ready and felt I could use a rest and was determined to have one.

Then there came the point when I knew I had to push, and I was using the squatting positions we had learnt in classes, my arms round my husband's neck, him holding me. The head kept popping in and out of view. And my goodness the down-breathing and chanting was so helpful. Then the baby (I still did not know the gender) was crowning, yes, I felt that ring of fire, but we all redoubled our breathing. Jen was beside me and, poor thing, I screamed at her 'sing, just SING!' and she did, and my husband joined in (badly, I imagine!), but they sang my lovely, beautiful daughter into the outside world. The midwife, an experienced Nigerian lady, was just there alongside, helping us out and keeping an eye, and I felt very looked after. Afterwards I felt so tired, but kind of glowing, basking in a mixture of happiness and relief like no other I had ever felt. And I had a daughter. She was born with a song, a gesture of love, generosity and creativity. Remarkable. All was well, and when I first looked at her, my heart had melted, and she looked back at me and, strange as it sounds, she looked so wise!

This little girl is now an adult, and she is living a life of song and adventure and love, continuing the pattern of her pregnancy and birth, and in fact is now planning to train to be a doula!

CHAPTER 11

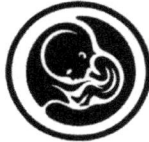

BIRTH, EMPOWERMENT, CHALLENGES, (AND IF UNLUCKY, TRAUMA)

This chapter tries to shed light on some of the challenges that can be encountered in the birth process and what we can learn from them. If I have learnt anything from interviewing so many women, it is that during pregnancy they generally do not want to hear too many difficult stories, so I apologise in advance for this section. However, it is also the case that forewarning can help, even when a birth does not go to plan. This chapter aims to think about how to make the best of challenges that can feel like curveballs, and to help women feel confident and empowered, in part by learning from examples of where things did not go as well as hoped. Take this example from Mia:

> *The birth of my first daughter was described by my midwife as a perfect textbook birth, but in fact I would describe it as a*

trauma. I had a perfect birth plan all written out (I am laughing at my own naivety now in thinking that I could control what happened). All went 'according to plan' with a water birth at the hospital birthing unit, but there was a miscommunication between me and the midwife during labour. I requested painkillers, and I didn't hear her say that she would see how the next contraction went and, if I still wanted them then, to ask again. She then put up a drip for fluids, and I mistakenly thought this was the drugs I had requested and continued with a very painful birth, thinking that these drugs were absolutely useless! When I discovered the mistake afterwards, I was furious but didn't have a chance to address it. I continued into serious post-natal depression, sometimes suicidal, and, needless to say, I struggled to bond with my baby.

Fast forward 21 months, and I was about to have my second child. I insisted on a C-section, and this time it was all smooth and I bonded instantly. No post-natal depression this time, the birth was calm, I recovered quickly.

I wonder to what extent the experience of the birth and the feelings of not being heard and emotionally held, or allowed to make the decisions that affected her, might have in turn affected her relationship with her infant. Mia had a bad experience this first time and needed to retake control the second time she gave birth, she did, and it worked.

Obviously, women want to give themselves the best chance of as smooth a birth as possible, not least to minimise pain and to increase the chances of nothing untoward happening to themselves or their baby. We also know that the quality of the experience of birth – for example, how traumatic it is – can have a knock-on effect on later mother-child relationships, as we saw in Mia's case. The research on postnatal stress and trauma symptoms testifies to this.[150] For example, mothers traumatised at birth can sometimes feel more rejecting of their babies, and in the worst cases, the mother-infant relationship can struggle to recover. This is an under-recognised phenomenon. When services and professionals are alert to the issues, and appropriate therapeutic support services are in place, we can avoid the worst effects.

In Maria's case, as she describes here, things did not go according to plan, but she and the mother-infant relationship recovered well:

> *When we arrived at the birthing centre, everything was prepared. There was a big birthing pool, my music was playing, and I felt calm again. The atmosphere was great. I briefly hesitated, as the midwife in charge was someone I had dealt with before, and I wasn't that fond of her.*
>
> *Against my will, they took us to the hospital. This turned the whole process around. I had written a letter that included what I wanted if it came to such an event. I asked my husband to give it to the hospital staff. I also told them a few things that would make the experience more comfortable. These included dimming the lights, having music playing, gift-giving to me by other women, my candle, letting me find out the sex myself, cutting the umbilical cord only after it had finished pumping, and putting the baby on my breast shortly before examining.*
>
> *Apart from the lights being dimmed, NONE of my requests were granted.*
>
> *I was in fear and pain and really dreaded the hospital once again. They forced open my waters; I got medication to progress the contractions and ended up having a caesarean with an epidural.*

They put the needle inside my spine during a contraction and held me down with four people. It didn't work, and they had to redo it. I was shaking by then.

When the baby was taken out, the physician screamed out that it was a boy. They didn't even show me the baby and took him away immediately. My husband was at least allowed to carry him under his shirt after he had been weighed and bathed. His APGAR score was all 10s. Fit and healthy.

Here, it was the loss of control that felt particularly bad, and the feeling of not being listened to, as well as not having the supportive midwife she had expected and wanted. In Maria's case, recovery was quick, in part because of her internal strength and the great support she had around her. This, though, is not so easy for all women, especially those who are less supported and less informed, and even more so for women from marginalised groups.

Sadly, a lot of the stress and even trauma around birth is avoidable, although we must remember that sometimes it is just down to pure bad luck. At the risk of sounding glib, probably the best way to work with birth trauma is to give oneself the best chance of preventing it. Many doulas and natural birth teachers argue strongly that when women are supported and empowered, then the chances of things going wrong reduce dramatically, even if the risks never go away. It is of course scary to give birth, more painful than any man like me can know, and some of the worst experiences come from a lack of control. Outcomes can be greatly influenced by the kinds of support and input received from those around them, whether midwives, doulas, or friends, or family.

Medical professionals generally have the best of intentions, but sometimes other agendas intrude and can disrupt a natural process. There can be a tendency to try to rush labour, even for as simple a reason as that it is time for doctors or midwives to change shifts. In such cases a woman's ability to trust their own bodies and to be supported in that can be undermined.

BBC radio host India Rakusen explained that:

> *There are occasions obviously within birth where it's like, this is definitely an emergency, and everyone needs to act. But I think that certainly there can be too many 'shoulds', and women are not always given the full picture of the risks and benefits, nor informed of all the options. It has definitely made me think differently about our next birth, and we're going to get a doula. And I've asked my sister and one of my best friends to be around for the birth.*

As well as the hands-on help that women should receive from a midwife and, if they are lucky, a doula, there is an awful lot of practical and emotional education that can help in the preparation for birth. This includes basics like what is the best position to be in to give birth and why. For most women, squatting and opening the pelvic outlet is preferable to, for example, lying on one's back. This makes more space for the baby and reduces the risk of tearing and other damage. Similarly, allowing a natural pause to rest between the stages of labour can be really helpful yet often be overridden by midwives and doctors. Valerie told me:

> *I had learnt that it was ok to pause and rest between the labour stages, before pushing, but I was really pressured to push even though I knew the baby wasn't ready. I wanted to trust my body and what I had been taught but did not want to upset the professionals. In the end, rather ridiculously, I actually pretended to be pushing, keeping a part of myself back to rest, but that was far from ideal.*

Similarly, the kinds of breathing and other techniques taught in hypnobirthing can reduce stress and tension and ease the process. Mindful birthing has helped many women realise that in the first stage of labour, women are experiencing contractions less than a quarter of the time, and the experience of birth can be greatly helped if they are supported to find ways to relax and replenish between contractions, rather than tensing in anxiety against the next one.

Information and advocacy

Women in labour can often be helped by what the medical profession might not always encourage, which is advocacy by a supportive birth partner. As experienced doula, Nikita Akilapa, reminded me, while doctors have real and much-needed expertise, they rarely witness a natural birth because, as senior medics, they tend to only be called in if things look to be going wrong. Rather, it is people like midwives, doulas, and active birth teachers, who have more experience of 'physiological births', who can best help to advocate for mothers. As Nikita told me:

> *If you have alternative information, you can go to your care team, to your doctor, or your midwife and argue for what you want. But we don't always know where to get that information. Sometimes medical staff leave it right to the very end to have important conversations, when you're really close to giving birth. And then they'll say, oh no, because you've got x, you can't do Y (e.g. have a home birth or the birth centre). Up until that point, you may have mentioned that you want the birth centre, and they'll say, oh yeah, well, we'll talk about that in week 36, knowing that it's likely that the protocol would mean saying no, you can't have it.*

Many people, especially those who don't have support, such as from a doula, will be disappointed but go along with the 'experts'. It can help if someone asks, 'Can you provide me with the data that tells you it's unsafe for me to have the birth centre?' And once they've presented it to you, you can then see if there is another possible set of data.

In the UK there are organisations such as Aims or Birthrights, who can help to access data in a bite-size format so it's easy for you to digest. You can even just call them and explain the issue and they'll compile an email for you with all of the relevant legal information, finding all of the right medical research.

I have heard the head of midwifery say things like 'say, you're right. So, let's now talk about how we give you access to the birth centre. We'll let you go on there if you agree to have a managed third stage, which is the synthetic oxytocin injection, to reduce the risk of bleeding, because someone with fibroids has a slightly higher risk of haemorrhaging in the postpartum. And we'd like you to have a cannula put in before you go into the birth centre. If you agree to those things, the birth centre is yours.'

Women in labour can often be helped by advocacy from a supportive knowledgeable birth partner, obviously preferably done in a way that gets the medical team onside rather than alienating them.

Trauma can happen anyway, through bad luck, but it is surprising how much can be prevented with the help of those who are expert in the birth process. Until recently the main traumas people were aware of were of physical or medical complications, which can be terrifying and leave women with their lives at risk. However, the psychological aspects of a traumatic birth have recently been receiving more attention.

In more serious cases this can tip into what is called obstetric violence. The kinds of things we need to help women watch out for and not accept include verbal abuse, unwanted touch (especially with sexual connotations), and intervening without proper consent. An Australian researcher[151] interviewed over 8,000 women, and some of the key themes in relation to obstetric violence include feeling dehumanised, violated, powerless, and, for example, being treated as a 'number' or 'object'. This chapter, and book, are meant to empower, not alarm, readers, and that is why having an advocate who is well prepared can be so important. Equally, it is important to be prepared to walk a tricky tightrope, to try to keep as much control of the process as possible by being involved in decisions, but also to have the flexibility to go with the unexpected where necessary.

International samples suggest that there is a much higher rate of PTSD than there should be after birth,[152] which, in turn, can contribute to a range of other issues in the postpartum period, both for the baby and also for the mother, such as less good feeding, sleep, or bonding. Many mothers describe how they were paid little attention after a traumatic birth. Researchers such as Emma Svanberg have described how doctors and health visitors and others often suggest that, even if the birth was traumatic, if the baby is fine, then mothers should be grateful. The traumatised women's own issues get lost in this process.[153] Svanberg likens this to being in a car accident and people only being interested in whether the car is ok! Of course, the health and safety of the baby are paramount, but few babies will thrive if the person looking after them is in a traumatised state. Much could be done to reduce the risk of birth trauma generally and obstetric violence in particular, and screening can be important here. For professionals or pregnant people reading this, a history of early trauma, and especially sexual abuse, is an important risk factor and so also a reason to get extra support as well as inner resolve, if possible.

Here is Anne's account of her experience giving birth to twins:

> *Standard NHS protocols meant that I was advised to be induced when we reached 36 weeks. In hindsight, with what I know now, I would have requested daily monitoring instead and waited for labour to begin naturally. But at the time I had concerns about twin 2 (T2, as they get labelled on scans), as I couldn't feel her movements so much. Twin 1, who by now was on the left-hand side, was frequently lively and left me in no doubt about her presence. Twin 2 was on the right, and there were long gaps with no distinct movement from her. I felt she would be safer on the outside than on the inside. So, the induction went ahead, and there began a difficult two days of labour.*

> *I had to stay in hospital alone and felt frightened and lonely when my waters broke during the night. A midwife came to do an internal check, which was agony; her manner was rough and unapologetic. The next morning, I was put on a drip to speed the contractions up, and had an epidural, which mostly worked, but not entirely, so there was a section of my uterus that felt the strength and pain of each contraction. Apparently for much of the remainder of the labour, I was not really with it, so it was mainly my husband enduring the anxiety and uncertainty of twin 1's heartbeat dropping during contractions, and the labour not progressing as it should. He phoned his sister, a GP, and she phoned a consultant, who came sweeping into the room and changed the care plan, sending me to the operating theatre to have a spinal block and a forceps-assisted delivery. The staff in there were very kind and reassuring, and, before too long, twin*

> *1 was safely delivered and placed on my partner's chest, and twin number two followed three minutes later, and was placed on my chest.*

This was a difficult experience but not overtly violent or abusive, and Anne was lucky to have what not many people have, a GP as a sister-in-law who could fight her corner. Even so, such experiences can leave a legacy, and Anne's example shows again the importance of knowledgeable advocates.

In the worst cases, some forms of obstetric trauma should be seen as yet another form of gendered violence. The British Birth Trauma Association give a figure of around 5% of women who suffer from actual PTSD symptoms; in fact, some people suggest that the figure is much higher. This is all the more reason to argue that women need to be helped to become more empowered in the birth process.

India Rakusen told me:

> *We were really lucky in that nothing was traumatic for the baby, and nothing was really traumatic for me. But he was induced at 42 plus two and we pushed back on that induction again and again and again, but to the point where I was like, let's just do it because I'm so anxious now. The word stillbirth has been said to me so many times, I can't bear this. But I look back and I just think, a bit more digging and a bit more support from someone, and I probably would have gone for foetal monitoring. And that was a real option, because he was so fine all the way through. Then there was this gruelling, horrible three-day-long induction, which ended in a caesarean section anyway.*
>
> *It's the lack of control that's most difficult. I called a pregnancy yoga teacher, and the most helpful thing she said was that you are as responsible for this baby. now, as you are when it's born.*

But it doesn't always work out like that. I was looking to everyone else, what should I do? And she just went, you are responsible for this baby right now. Positivity can be great, but you need to know all of the possible options and what they could look like.

So once again we see the importance of women having information, control, and choice, as well as good emotional and expert support.

Many of the more difficult stories in this guide have featured induction, and again a central issue seems to be, if things are not going to plan, how uninformed women are and how little choice they feel they have, and, most importantly, as leading midwives such as campaigner, author, and expert midwife Sarah Wickham have long argued,[154] who the decision is being made for. Wickham suggests that many of the procedures are designed to ensure quick, efficient, and safe delivery, but this might not take account of the experiences and needs of the women giving birth. Interestingly, it might not take account of the baby's choices either. What are called spontaneous births, as opposed to induction or C-section, are often less than 50% of total births now, at least in the United Kingdom, and in fact even less than that in some countries. However, much research suggests that the birth is not so much 'spontaneous' as led by the baby when it is ready. Such 'spontaneous' births do have many benefits, including the release of a massive cocktail of hormones that reduce pain, ease the passage, and have a host of other beneficial effects, some long-lasting.

Inductions can sometimes be lifesaving and are generally advised for the best of reasons. But as senior midwife Scarlett Granville told me:

> *This is a huge and complicated subject, especially the questions about who and why and when we induce, the way we talk to women about induction, the methods and cascade of interventions that follow, the environment in which inductions are started (too often a ward, not a private room). All these and other factors have a significant impact on outcomes and on women's experiences, many of which are negative. This can affect the mode of birth, the extent of blood loss, the interruption of skin-to-skin contact and the establishment of breastfeeding; the pain felt in labour, the increased anxiety, and lack of control from poor communication also affect the length of stay in busy postnatal wards, as well as the rates of post-natal depression and post-natal bonding.*
>
> *Rates of induction are now 30–50% in the UK. This is done with the good intention of reducing stillbirth rates and neonatal morbidity. In the UK there's a national target for maternity services, but ultimately it is just not done in a way that is woman-focused, and as a result women and babies sometimes pay a heavy price.*

It is often after difficult birth experiences that postnatal depression is diagnosed when in reality what we are seeing are the effects of birth trauma. It is interesting that after reading this Karina Sarmiento, a perinatal parenting expert, told me that she could recall hardly any cases of women who had had a doula during the birth coming to her services. I suspect this is not always true, but nonetheless getting good prenatal and birth support is a powerful preventative measure. It is quite clear that, as in so many traumatic experiences, feeling out of control, or being given interventions that are not chosen or desired, can be a trigger. Not surprisingly, women who already have a background of traumatic experiences, and especially women who have experienced sexual abuse, are more susceptible to feeling traumatised.

There are many lessons to be learnt still, but some of the key take-home messages include that prenatal education is really important, that support makes a huge difference, as does skilled advocacy, and that, where possible, it is important to help women to feel in a position to make informed decisions and to consent and be in control of their own process. Birth is obviously a very personal experience, and although there are technocratic aspects to it, what is hoped for is to create an atmosphere in which women are listened to, taken seriously, and able to access the support they choose, and that birthing services are trauma-informed and organised in as compassionate way as possible.

Some lessons from less easy births

As many of the guides in this series will attest, a good start is not essential to a child's mental health, but it certainly helps. A good birth increases the chances of laying better emotional foundations, and the chances of a smooth birth are enhanced by having good support. Equally, the capacity to bond well with a baby is increased when mothers feel emotionally safe and cared for, which, in turn, reduces the risk of other problems, such as postnatal depression.[155] Debbie's story sheds light on this:

> *The last few weeks of my pregnancy 'went south', with a sinus infection resulting in a prescription of painkillers which I reacted to by coming out in a rash over my pregnant bump and chest. I was due in two weeks. How would I give birth? I hadn't slept in over a week. My mum arrived to my rescue. I began to relax but went into labour a week early. I began labour, and it*

progressed quickly. A difficult but natural delivery. I struggled to give birth. I later learned my baby was 'back-to-back'. A boy. Enormous. Bald. I was expecting a girl. Or else another tiny dark hairy boy. Exhausted, I crawled into bed, having given birth downstairs. It all seemed surreal. My new huge baby in a basket next to me. My older baby came home in his pyjamas and burst through the door to see me and meet his brother. I just didn't have the energy for either baby.

'I can't', I said. 'You have to', replied my mum. So I pretended. I pretended for weeks, for months. I felt nothing. Nothing except loss. Loss for my baby in his pyjamas. I didn't know I would have to say goodbye to him and what we had together. My perfect, tiny, dark-haired little baby who had arrived like a breath of fresh air following the sudden death of his paternal grandad. Assumptions were made. About my confidence and my capacity to mother. I wonder if this was because I had chosen to give birth at home. The first seven months were hell. My new baby responded to my lack of connection with skin irritation (eczema) and voracious bowl movements (at least seven times a day). I know now it must have been so hard for him. It was not the best start for either of us. We feel it still. It was 16 years ago.

This is a mother who needed much more understanding and support than she received, and such support and the experience of being advocated for is what badly needs to be fought for.

One factor that professionals, such as midwives, as well as parents and partners, could be more alert to is the impact of a parent's own childhood trauma on the birth process. For example, one recent large study[156] found that a pregnant mother's own history of trauma, especially emotional abuse and neglect, was strongly correlated with a fear of childbirth.

If one is a member of a discriminated-against group, such as being a black person in a more racist society, then this in itself can have serious consequences. Nikita Akilapa told me:

> *Some people can have a more challenging experience navigating the system simply because of the colour of their skin, and women of colour can receive less compassionate and vigilant perinatal care. For example, many of my clients have been threatened with social services in a bid to deter them from leaving before officially being discharged. In my experience, this happens far more often to black and brown women, than any other group. In one such case my client, an African American woman, was desperate to leave the postnatal ward. These wards are notoriously busy and loud, and she was struggling to rest and breastfeed there. As this was her second child, she knew she'd be better off at home, in a more oxytocin-friendly environment. When she asked to leave, she was threatened with social services. She was warned that leaving before official discharge creates a safeguarding issue … even though the baby was only waiting on a hearing test, and mum had offered to return as an outpatient the following day. Unbeknownst to the midwife, my client is actually a lawyer who writes hospital policies. Upon learning this, and on meeting her white husband, the midwife quickly backtracked on the threat. My client actually plans to create a 'fact and action' pack for women who are at risk of encountering this sort of treatment!*

In fact, shockingly, in the United Kingdom black women are as much as four times more likely to experience serious and even life-threatening complications in childbirth than white women[157] – a terrible statistic. Indeed, we see the same in the United States and in some other countries.[158] Black women are also more likely to report mistreatment and neglect from providers and to experience trauma around the birth.[159]

We have already heard from Arya, a care-experienced black woman, about frankly neglectful experiences, underlining just how different the process can be both if one has a background of trauma and also if one is a woman of colour:

> *The midwife announced that she would fetch the doctor, as my baby's heart rate has gone up, and then they gave me an episiotomy without my permission and forcepped my child out. It was extremely traumatic. Following this, I was put into a room with other mums and told that I should mix feed, as he was so little. I said I wanted to breastfeed, but this was ignored.*

> *The midwife who later saw me at home was shocked by what had happened. We then had to spend a week in hospital, as my baby had to have phototherapy for jaundice. He was put in a box naked, with an eye mask. I was not allowed to take him out unless to feed him every three hours. He cried, and I could not bear that and took him out. The only time the midwives came to check was to tell me off for doing that. I was on my own on a ward with other screaming babies. I had no sleep, no support at my most vulnerable time. My husband was only allowed to come during visiting times, and so I had no help at all. With no family to advocate on my behalf, it was so difficult. No one showed me things like where the shower was, or where and when to get food.*

> *Being a care-experienced person, for my whole life I had no one to depend on, so asking for help was not on my radar. With hindsight I would have spent money on a doula, someone who would advocate for me and be my voice. I think my difficult experiences were absolutely linked with my ethnicity, an Indian woman who was quiet and compliant; and it also reactivated many painful early losses. I found these early months so very difficult and could not reach out for help because I felt I would be judged.*

Arya clearly needed someone like Nikita to advocate for her! On hearing Arya's story, Nikita told me:

> *Unfortunately, it happens too frequently that women of colour are dismissed, not listened to or believed, treated uncompassionately. If a woman feels uncomfortable with her care team because of her antenatal treatment, how will that impact on her feelings of safety at birth? If trauma is sustained at birth, what are the chances of a mother reaching out to the NHS for any necessary postnatal support – be it for breastfeeding or mental health? The repercussions of this can be long-lasting for the entire family.*

And we know that the higher the anxiety, the greater the likelihood of a difficult labour. A recurring theme in this and the other guides is the importance of psychological and emotional support. Screening and looking out for often hidden historical trauma can make a big difference. A history of sexual abuse perhaps more than anything needs to be taken seriously, as for such women, the birth process can be much more triggering and needs to be handled with immense sensitivity.

Sometimes just plain bad luck intrudes into the birth process, including physiological complications, and at the risk of repeating a kind of mantra, it is always important for there to be as little blame as possible when things do go wrong. As Jessica James reminded me:

> *What I've learned over the years, it's not the type of birth you have that leaves you traumatised. It's the way it was handled and the way you felt, the extent to which you understood what went on and the amount of control over how it went, but also how informed one is. You might unexpectedly need to have a caesarean and feel absolutely fine about it because you*

understood why and were involved in the decision. What's really traumatic is when something's done to you and you feel completely out of control and you don't really understand. Interestingly, some women have what sounded like the most horrendous birth in terms of the actual facts of it. It took hours. They tried to do this, and they couldn't do it. And then they did that, and then, you know, they went through everything, but they feel, well, we really worked at it. We really did our best. Its most important that women feel 'you did your best'. It can be a disaster if someone is told that if you do what I tell you, then it's all going to be all right.

Here is Maria who we met before:

One day after the calculated birth date the baby wanted to make its way to the earth. I dilated 10 centimetres at home, with my husband supporting me. The waters never broke, but I didn't think about it.

I breathed into the contractions, which were intense but were very manageable, and I have very fond memories of this phase. I wasn't scared at all and felt very confident. The contractions felt like powerful waves. I connected to the baby.

After about nine hours we called the midwife on duty. She arrived with a colleague. I had never seen her or the other one before. She was very friendly and amazed that I had done 10 centimetres on my own. I overheard a conversation with a midwife I knew, who could not come. I found it strange. I quickly thought, if I asked for a house birth, which was an option with the birthing centre as I felt calm and good at home and knew the drive to the centre would interrupt that flow. I don't know why, but I went into the car with my husband next to me, and one the midwives. In the car journey was the first time I found the contractions painful.

The birth slowed down once I was in the pool. The midwife tried to turn the baby's head during one of the contractions, and that is when its heartrate dropped. I had to go to the foetal monitor and that interrupted my breathing routine, and I also had to lie on the side, which felt very uncomfortable. After about five minutes the midwife decided to bring me to the hospital next-door. I begged her not to, but I was dilated for too long, and she didn't dare to do otherwise. It is important that we as women still go for what we want, whether water births or whatever, but it is also important to try to not feel bad or guilty if things take another course.

In Maria's case we see how bad luck can intrude, but we are left wondering about the effects of a few possible miscalculations and, perhaps more importantly, the effect of the absence of the supportive person whom she had been expecting. In general, research suggests that psychological, social, and biological factors interact; reducing stress levels through emotional support and good advocacy by experienced birthing professionals and, very importantly, good prenatal preparation leads, on average at least, to healthier pregnancies, easier labours, fewer birth complications, and seemingly better outcomes generally. But we can never predict what will happen, and, as Maria said:

When being asked how I felt, I just repeated the sentence 'I am in the here and now.'

Being in the 'here and now' and accepting whatever happens is not, by any means, easy but seems a pretty good place to aim for, in fact one that Maria mostly managed. I recently met her lovely, sensitive, and strong little two-year-old who is adorable, and the whole family are doing very well. When things go wrong, it needn't be a disaster, but we also must not underestimate the potential adverse consequences of such difficult experiences, and hence the need to educate and advocate and ensure the highest level of support.

Here's Nikita again, with a hopeful story:

> *One client was pregnant with her second baby. Her first birth had been very medically managed and had left her feeling quite traumatised. She was far more vigilant this time about obstetric violence and medical coercion. She wanted to be prepared and hired me for antenatal education, birth support, and advocacy.*
>
> *She felt she was not being listened to at her hospital – she had fibroids and wasn't allowed to use the birth centre. Although her consultant at the hospital had signed her off for a non-medical birth on the birth centre, the Head of Midwifery was not in agreement. Despite calling in expert services for support, there was no flexibility. This dismissiveness eventually turned into what felt like coercion, when she was told her baby was going to be too big for a vaginal birth anyway, and she'd need to be induced at 40 weeks. She took herself to another trust, but bizarrely, this time they said her baby was too small, and they were keen to induce labour in case there was a problem with her placenta.*
>
> *This mother was in touch with her body and baby, and she instinctively knew all was well and fought not to have an induction. I connected her with an independent midwife for a consultation, including a risk assessment of her circumstances, and medical reassurance around her preferences. This, plus her antenatal education and unwavering support from her husband, gave her confidence to hold her ground.*
>
> *When she went into labour, she actually felt much safer staying at home with just her husband and myself. After a short labour she successfully free-birthed at home. Her baby was about 7.5 lb. Not too big, not too small! She went to hospital after*

her freebirth for some suturing, and it was confirmed that her placenta was healthy.

Without a doula, this would have been a very different birth experience.

Hopefully most women are not faced with having to fight the system. However, this example shows once again what a huge difference both support and information can make. Ideally, one would not want to ever antagonise a hospital team, but too many women can be easily persuaded by statements about danger, and they can lack the confidence to trust their bodies and to find out the information they need to assert their rights.

The lessons from these birth chapters are similar to those in the whole book and, indeed, the series. Mothers and children, and any of us, need to feel supported, cared for, and, indeed, loved. We need to know that someone has our back and that we can rely on others with more experience than ourselves, who can fight for us and deeply hold us in mind. Blame and, worse, self-blame, are unhelpful and make things worse.

Things do not always go to plan, and so we cannot afford to be too rigid. Knowledge and advocacy help, so we are not passive recipients of medical and other systems and can reclaim as much agency as we can. Mothers and babies, and indeed all humans, need communities which are caring, supportive, and, indeed, open-hearted. Everything is easier when we feel loved, when the oxytocin is flowing, when we do not contract or tense out of fear or stress but can be open to possibility. We need to feel safe for that to happen.

EPILOGUE

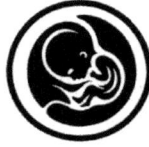

Life in the womb and life with a life in one's womb

Thank you for joining me on what I hope has been a fascinating journey, even if it evoked both excitement and some trepidation. We certainly have seen that life in the womb, like all life, is complex, full of challenges, but most importantly, has extraordinary potential. I have deliberately not shirked the challenges, mainly because, when we know about potential dangers, generally we can do things to mitigate the risks. As research[81] and clinical work have consistently shown, pregnancy is indeed a period of risk, but also of adaptation and with the potential for developing genuine resilience. In other words, we know now that we can make a huge difference to later outcomes when we have the right information. intrauterine environment.

I started by looking at many of the most fascinating facts about what happens after conception right through to the time of birth. We saw what an amazing being the foetus is, with surprising abilities to get what it needs, to actively interact with its mother, able to do so many things we might not have thought possible so early in its existence. A central theme has been that the unborn baby is both an autonomous being but also is totally dependent, it is learning about the world it is

140

likely to come into, adapting to it, and responding to signals it is picking up from its unique intrauterine environment.

I thought about bonding, about what we can learn from ultrasound scans, and we saw how the foetal brain and its millions of brain cells enable some incredible mental capacities to come online well before birth. Some of you might have been surprised by the slightly left-field topic of prenatal bonding, but I hope I have persuaded you that such bonding can set the foundations for good, attuned, and loving later experiences. The themes of bonding echo others in the book: that it is good loving emotional connection, trust and ease, that leads to emotional and physical health.

I hope I have taken seriously the importance of culture and how non-Western or non-WEIRD models and indigenous knowledge can offer us so much, indeed much that we have lost, despite the very real gains of Western science. We saw that in many cultures, the processes of pregnancy and birth are imbued with ancient rituals, a spiritual heart, and occurs with the support of experienced elders. While infant mortality has lessened with modern healthcare, possibly something has also been lost in the transition to medical hospital-based models, not least ancient socio-spiritual rituals. Being held by traditional ways has many knock-on effects, not least very real benefits for the nervous systems of the mother, and hence also the foetus, that come with a deep sense of belonging.

Our journey has not all been about love and ease. We have seen how there can be complex ambivalent feelings about having a baby, and that difficult feelings should be expected. In fact, we saw how conflict is inevitable, indeed right down to the cellular level, such as between the paternal and maternal genome or between the mother's and baby's needs. Both the unborn baby and birthgiver are sharing, and sometimes competing for, space and resources. What we see is very much co-embodiment and with luck, co-regulation, but always a two-way interaction which also includes some competition.

I have tried to avoid either blame or guilt and have suggested that, rather than it all being down to the parents, an unborn baby can pay a price for what happened in previous generations. Every foetus, indeed, every one of us, is a product of our intergenerational inheritances, including our socio-economic, cultural, genetic, and epigenetic history, as well as current influences. We saw that when a parent has had more adverse childhood experiences, there is more risk to their children's long-term health outcomes.[3] There is no room for blame, as adverse experiences such as poverty, racism, and intergenerational trauma are so out of the control of people experiencing them.

I hope I have similarly avoided guilt by pointing out the need for healthy vigilance about potential dangers from a pregnant person being exposed to certain substances such as some drugs, alcohol as well as too much stress, and pollutants, but we should still be aware of a foetus's sensitivity. It is extraordinary to see how this bundle of cells is continually receiving biochemical and other feedback and adapting and responding to this. As quoted earlier from researcher David Chamberlain, 'the womb is the first school of life'.[5]

And this took us to the final chapters where stories from many women helped us to learn about the actual process of birth. So much about this, and later guides, centres on the importance of women being supported enough to feel safe and at ease, to be helped to know and listen to their bodies and to be given the right information. In birth as in so much else in life, women often need help to make sense of what and who to trust, to get the right balance between trusting their

142

own bodies, their intuition and sense of what her baby needs, alongside medical expertise, expectations, and procedures.

Throughout the book, I have highlighted the vital importance of support from others, whether partners, friends, or experienced women such as doulas. Good social connection and feeling safe are essential for human psychological health, perhaps never more so than for a new mother. Stress and fear, the opposite of feeling safe, can lead to tensing, a drawing inward, away from trust and openness, just when we need them most. What I hope is clear from this book is how much we now know about how to maximise the likelihood of good experiences and optimal outcomes, to give the unborn baby the very best chance of their best life.

A central message has been that, well before birth, we see a being who is already learning, making predictions, adapting to its unique environment, but has its own agenda. We might not be able to change a parent's past, but we can have a big impact on the current environment that the foetus is adapting to. We hope that as many new babies as possible are born as little beings who already expect, in their very cells and nascent psyches, that the world they will experience will be one of love, trust, safeness, and hopefully, joy. We know now that when we build good foundations then outcomes tend to be so much better.

And when they are born: what next?

Then the meeting of the little one – a fanfare is needed here – an absolutely unworldly, strange, familiar and yet disappointingly unexpected and excruciatingly marvellous sight. A reconciliation must be made: this is both who and not who I have been speaking with all this time. This is now not me, this is novel, this is the beginning of something new, and my mind is blown and my body is infused with the most glorious high, and wow, I'm exhausted, and what have I done? This is actually real! (Emily)

Now the adventure really begins, one that is often challenging and, if we are lucky, exhilarating and life-enhancing. I have written a lot about the importance of both practical and emotional support, which makes bonding and parenting so much easier. This can be especially the case when a birth is difficult. So many new mothers talk about the relief of having the support of both experienced older women who have already been through this, as well as of other new mothers who are sharing similar issues. Indeed, other new mothers might be the only people who show any interest in things like the colour of a baby's pooh, nappy rash, or feeding techniques. It's a time when ordinary support and friendships between mothers can really pay dividends. One mother told me of her gratitude when a neighbour brought some food around, while another woman, who had had a difficult relationship with her father, was amazed when he brought her sanitary pads after the birth, which she needed; this was a rare expression of fathering – an experience of a loving hand from him that she had always longed for and had rarely received.

One mother, Valerie, described the delicacy of the new intimacy:

To begin with after the birth, I felt a total attunement with my child, as though I knew her completely and she me. We could read each other totally. The idea of needing to talk to communicate seemed alien. Why would this be necessary? She already knew what I was thinking and I her, words would only get in the way? Communication using speech was a painful reminder that we were now separate and our attachment, once

144

so completely intimate, was now changed.

Yet it is often not an easy time. We hear in the second guide about postnatal depression, for example. Many mothers describe how their own traumatic childhoods get in the way of being with their baby in a relaxed way. Sally told me:

> *When my son was born after three days of labour, I had a terrible and irrational fear that he would be taken from me. It was as though he had always existed for me. Such was my fear that I used the tie from my dressing gown and attached one end to my wrist and the other to my son's ankle. I now understand this fear of loss and where it came from so well, but at the time it seemed perfectly reasonable to me. It was real. The nurses wanted to put him in a separate ward with the other babies so the mothers could sleep, but of course I refused. I was called 'selfish' and I was, self-ish. But I was also in love.*

Life outside the womb opens the door to new worlds and possibilities, and this is the subject of the next guide in the series. Here we learn how the human infant is born extremely immature and can do little unaided in its first months. Its survival requires fairly constant physical and emotional care. We see how babies are born pre-wired with extraordinarily impressive capacities for social interaction. They can elicit the human responses they need to survive and thrive and are born with an incredible ability to respond to the social environments in which they find themselves.

Infants are especially born wired to relate, and to recognise and respond to their mother's smells, voice, and gestures, from birth onwards. They actively adapt to their social environment, learning both what to expect from it and how to actively influence it. We will see how bonding is gradual and not guaranteed, and rejection of infants has not been uncommon in human history. We see how luckier infants receive attuned attention, but that not all do, and that this depends on levels of parental support and a parent's own history and psychology. We see how newborns maximise their attractiveness, such as features of 'babyness', to survive, including large heads, big eyes, round faces, prominent foreheads, which all tend to induce positive and protective feelings and deter aggression.

We see how even newborn babies are already able to recognise faces, smells, and sounds and become acculturated, whether to the rhythms of an African hunter-gatherer tribe or a Western European middle-class family. A baby can be like a sponge for emotional, psychological, or cultural atmospheres, picking up and adapting to moods and emotional expectations. Infants 'entrain' to the rhythms of their environment, and in microsecond encounters are learning expectable behaviour patterns – whether a highly interactive or a more socially withdrawn one. All infants are learning to survive and thrive in the particular world in which they find themselves, using the hugely varied stock of responses with which evolution has endowed them.

In short, in the next guide you will see how babies arrive with very wide-ranging potential, while the ways in which adults respond to babies vary enormously and make a huge difference to how this potential gets expressed. A central lesson of this guide on prenatal life, and of the next guide and all the others, is that human life develops from the delicate interplay of nature and nurture, a bundle of inherited potentials meeting with the cultural, social, and personal influences of the adults in an infant's life. I hope this exciting idea, and the information in these guides can help in a small way to optimise the chances of a healthy, happy, and easeful start to life.

146

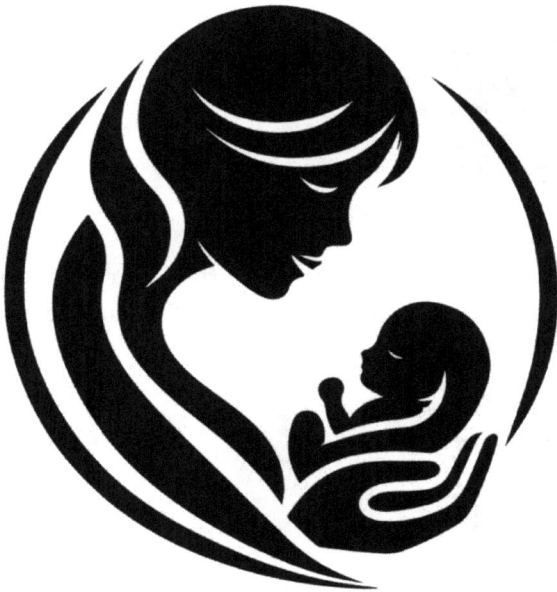

Thank you for reading Womb Life by Dr. Graham Music.

If you enjoyed this, please sign up for Graham Music's newsletter, which includes new blogs, and news on publications, and forthcoming events *here* or using this QR code

Find out more about his work from his website *https://nurturingnatures.co.uk/* or click on this barcode to access it:

You can also find his online courses on many child development, clinical and neuroscience subjects *here*, *https://graham-s-site-453c.thinkific.com/collections*, or access them by using this barcode

Graham can be contacted via the website, or by email, gmusic@nurturingnatures.co.uk, or link with him on social media such as twitter/X (@grahammusic1), or LinkedIn (*www.linkedin.com/in/graham-music-nurturing-natures*).

Finally, it really makes more difference to authors than you might think, so PLEASE consider leaving a review on any site you use, such as Amazon, BookBub or Goodreads.

Below are Graham Music's other books:

Music, G (2022) Respark: Igniting Hope and Joy after Trauma and Depression . London: Mind-Nurturing Books

Music, G. (2022, 2001) Affect and Emotions: A Brief Psychoanalytic Tour London: Mind-Nurturing Books

Music, G. (2024/2016/2010) Nurturing Natures: Attachment and Children's Emotional, Social and Brain Development (3nd edition) | London: Psychology Press

Music, G (2019) | Nurturing Children: From Trauma to Growth using Attachment Theory, Psychoanalysis and Neurobiology | Oxford: Routledge

Music. G. (2014) | The Good Life: Wellbeing and the new science of Altruism, Selfishness and Immorality | Oxford: Routledge

And co-edited:

Nathanson, A; Music, G; Sternberg, J 2021 | From Trauma to Harming Others: Therapeutic Work with Delinquent, Violent and Sexually Harmful Children and Young People (2021) – Oxford: Routledge

REFERENCES

1. Waxman AG. Navajo childbirth in transition. Medical Anthropology. 1990 Mar 1;12(2):187–206.

2. Yehuda R, Lehrner A. Intergenerational transmission of trauma effects: putative role of epigenetic mechanisms. World Psychiatry. 2018;17(3):243–57.

3. Petruccelli K, Davis J, Berman T. Adverse childhood experiences and associated health outcomes: A systematic review and meta-analysis. Child Abuse & Neglect [Internet]. 2019 Nov 1;97

4. Bruner C. ACE, Place, Race, and Poverty: Building Hope for Children. Academic Pediatrics. 2017 Sep 1;17(7, Supplement):S123–9.

5. Chamberlain D. Windows to the Womb: Revealing the Conscious Baby from Conception to Birth. Berkeley,: North Atlantic Books; 2013.

6. Porges SW. Making the world safe for our children: Down-regulating defence and up-regulating social engagement to 'optimise' the human experience. Children Australia. 2015;40(2):114–23.

7. Ciaunica A, Constant A, Preissl H, Fotopoulou K. The first prior: From co-embodiment to co-homeostasis in early life. Consciousness and Cognition. 2021 May 1;91:103117.

8. Orloff NC, Hormes JM. Pickles and ice cream! Food cravings in pregnancy: hypotheses, preliminary evidence, and directions for future research. Front Psychol. 2014 Sep 23;5:1076.

9. Konlan KD, Abdulai JA, Konlan KD, Amoah RM, Doat A. Practices of pica among pregnant women in a tertiary healthcare facility in Ghana. Nurs Open. 2020 Jan 28;7(3):783–92.

10. Mistretta CM, Bradley RM. Taste and swallowing in utero: a discussion of fetal sensory function. British Medical Bulletin. 1975;31(1):80–4.

11. Sallenbach WB. The intelligent prenate: Paradigms in prenatal learning and bonding. In: Blum TP, editor. Prenatal Perception, Learning, and Bonding: learning and bonding. Hong Kong: Leonardo; 1993. p. 61–106.

12. Garcia-Faura A, Moens V, Lopez-Teijon M. EP27. 10: Fetal facial expression in response to intravaginal emission of different types of music. Ultrasound in Obstetrics & Gynecology. 2019;54:401–401.

13. Einspieler C, Prayer D, Marschik PB. Fetal movements: the origin of human behaviour. Developmental Medicine & Child Neurology. 2021;63(10):1142–8.

14. Goodlin R, Schmidt W. Human fetal arousal levels as indicated by heart rate recordings. Am J Obstet Gynecol. 1972;114(5):613–21.

15. Lucchini M, Shuffrey LC, Nugent JD, Pini N, Sania A, Shair M, et al. Effects of Prenatal Exposure to Alcohol and Smoking on Fetal Heart Rate and Movement Regulation. Frontiers in physiology. 2021;12.

16. Nordenstam F, Norman M, Wickström R. Blood pressure and heart rate variability in preschool children exposed to smokeless tobacco in fetal life. Journal of the

American Heart Association. 2019;8(21).

17. Derbyshire SW, Bockmann JC. Reconsidering fetal pain. Journal of Medical Ethics. 2020 Jan 1;46(1):3–6.

18. Krueger C, Garvan C. Cardiac orienting to auditory stimulation in the fetus. SAGE Open Nursing. 2019;5:1–15.

19. Almas YM, Santhosh M, Bryant J. Prenatal programming-potential modulator for development of personality, preferences and skills. International Journal of Advanced Research in Medicine. 2022;(4 (1)):164–8.

20. Ustun B, Reissland N, Covey J, Schaal B, Blissett J. Flavor Sensing in Utero and Emerging Discriminative Behaviors in the Human Fetus. Psychol Sci. 2022 Oct 1;33(10):1651–63.

21. Dieter JNI, Emory EK, Johnson KC, Raynor BD. Maternal depression and anxiety effects on the human fetus: Preliminary findings and clinical implications. Infant Ment Health J. 2008 Sep 1;29(5):420–41.

22. Ogo K, Kanenishi K, Mori N, AboEllail MAM, Hata T. Change in fetal behavior in response to vibroacoustic stimulation. Journal of perinatal medicine. 2019;47(5):558–63.

23. Murray L, Cooper P, Fearon P. Parenting difficulties and postnatal depression: implications for primary healthcare assessment and intervention. Community Practitioner. 2014;87(11):34–8.

24. Piontelli A. From fetus to child: an observational and psychoanalytic study. London: Tavistock Publications; 1992.

25. Thomson-Salo F. Infant Observation: Creating Transformative Relationships. London: Karnac Books; 2014.

26. Hidas G, Raffai J, Vollner J. Prenatal Bonding Analysis: The Invisible Umbilical Cord. Oxford: Taylor & Francis; 2022.

27. Seong JS, Han YJ, Kim MH, Shim JY, Lee MY, Oh S young, et al. The risk of preterm birth in vanishing twin: A multicenter prospective cohort study. PLOS ONE. 2020 May 29;15(5):e0233097.

28. Dalton K. Intelligence and prenatal progesterone: A reappraisal. Vol. 72, Journal of the Royal Society of Medicine. SAGE Publications Sage UK: London, England; 1979.

29. Ganjeh BJ, Mirrafiei A, Jayedi A, Mirmohammadkhani M, Emadi A, Ehsani F, et al. The relationship between adherence to the Mediterranean dietary pattern during early pregnancy and behavioral, mood and cognitive development in children under 1 year of age: a prospective cohort study. Nutritional Neuroscience. 2023;0(0):1–8.

30. Barker D. Adult Consequences of Fetal Growth Restriction. Clinical Obstetrics & Gynecology. 2006;49(2):270.

31. Michońska I, Łuszczki E, Zielińska M, Oleksy Ł, Stolarczyk A, Dereń K. Nutritional Programming: History, Hypotheses, and the Role of Prenatal Factors in the Prevention of Metabolic Diseases-A Narrative Review. Nutrients. 2022 Oct 21;14(20):4422.

32. Ragusa A, Svelato A, Santacroce C, Catalano P, Notarstefano V, Carnevali O, et al. Plasticenta: First evidence of microplastics in human placenta. Environment International. 2021 Jan 1;146:106274.

33. Cunha YG de O, Amaral GCB do, Felix AA, Blumberg B, Amato AA. Early-life exposure to endocrine-disrupting chemicals and autistic traits in childhood and adolescence. Frontiers in Endocrinology [Internet]. 2023;14

34. Raffai J. Mother-child bonding-analysis in the prenatal realm: The strange events of a queer world. International Journal of Prenatal and Perinatal Psychology and Medicine. 1998;10:163–74.

35. Alyousefi-van Dijk K, De Waal N, Van IJzendoorn MH, Bakermans-Kranenburg MJ. Development and feasibility of the prenatal video-feedback intervention to promote positive parenting for expectant fathers. J Reprod Infant Psychol. 2022 Sep;40(4):352–65.

36. Bowlby J. Attachment and loss. Vol. 1, Attachment. London: Hogarth; 1969.

37. Hrdy SB. Mother nature: Maternal instincts and how they shape the human species. London: Chatto & Windus; 2000.

38. Tronick EZ, Morelli GA, Winn S. Multiple Caretaking of Efe (Pygmy) Infants. American Anthropologist. 1987;89(1):96–106.

39. Benedek T. Parenthood as a developmental phase: A contribution to the libido theory. Journal of the American psychoanalytic Association. 1959;7(3):389–417.

40. Deutch H. The psychology of women: a psychoanalytic interpretation (Vol. 2). New York Gurne and Stratton. 1945;

41. Rubin R. Maternal tasks in pregnancy. Maternal-Child Nursing Journal. 1975;4(3):143.

42. Lumley JM. Attitudes to the fetus among primigravidae. Journal of Paediatrics and Child Health. 1982;18(2):106–9.

43. Tichelman E, Westerneng M, Witteveen AB, Baar AL van, Horst HE van der, Jonge A de, et al. Correlates of prenatal and postnatal mother-to-infant bonding quality: A systematic review. PLOS ONE. 2019 Sep 24;14(9):e0222998.

44. Cranley MS. The Origins of the Mother-Child Relationshp-A Review. Physical & Occupational Therapy in Pediatrics. 1993;12(2–3):39–51.

45. Condon JT. The assessment of antenatal emotional attachment: Development of a questionnaire instrument. British Journal of Medical Psychology. 1993;66(2):167–83.

46. Appleton K, Atluru A. Maternal-Fetal Bonding: Ultrasound Imaging's Role in enhancing This Important Relationship. Donald School Journal of Ultrasound in Obstetrics and Gynecology. 2012 Dec 1;6(4):408–11.

47. Stone NI, Downe S, Dykes F, Rothman BK. "Putting the baby back in the body": The re-embodiment of pregnancy to enhance safety in a free-standing birth center. Midwifery. 2022 Jan;104:103172.

48. Zeanah CH, Carr S, Wolk S. Fetal movements and the imagined baby of pregnancy: Are they related? Journal of Reproductive and Infant Psychology. 1990;8(1):23–36.

49. Brandon AR, Pitts S, Denton WH, Stringer CA, Evans HM. A history of the theory of prenatal attachment. J Prenat Perinat Psychol Health. 2009;23(4):201–22.

50. Pollock PH, Percy A. Maternal antenatal attachment style and potential fetal abuse. Child Abuse & Neglect. 1999;23(12):1345–57.

51. Zehra S, Sharma DC. Impact of Music Therapy on Fetus and Mother by sonography. In 2023.

52. Pino O, Di Pietro S, Poli D. Effect of Musical Stimulation on Placental Programming and Neurodevelopment Outcome of Preterm Infants: A Systematic Review. International Journal of Environmental Research and Public Health. 2023 Jan;20(3):2718.

53. Hüther G. The significance of exposure to music for the formation and stabilisation of complex neuronal relationship matrices in the human brain: In: Music that works: Contributions of biology, neurophysiology, psychology, sociology, medicine and musicology. Springer; 2009. p. 119–30.

54. Nagy E, Thompson P, Mayor L, Doughty H. Do foetuses communicate? Foetal responses to interactive versus non-interactive maternal voice and touch: An exploratory analysis. Infant Behavior and Development. 2021 May 1;63:101562.

55. Gottlieb A. The afterlife is where we come from: The culture of infancy in West Africa. Chicago: University of Chicago Press; 2004.

56. Putnam RD. Bowling alone: The collapse and revival of American community. New York: Simon & Schuster; 2000.

57. Hari J. Lost Connections: Uncovering the Real Causes of Depression – and the Unexpected Solutions. Bloomsbury Publishing; 2018.

58. Rachmayanti RD, Diana R, Anwar F, Khomsan A, Riyadi H, Christianti DF, et al. Culture, traditional beliefs and practices during pregnancy among the Madurese tribe in Indonesia. British Journal of Midwifery. 2023 Mar 2;31(3):148–56.

59. Klein M. Notes on some schizoid mechanisms. International Journal of Psycho-Analysis. 1946;27:99–110.

60. Trivers R. Natural selection and social theory: selected papers of Robert L. Trivers. Oxford: Oxford University Press; 2002.

61. Pritschet L, Taylor CM, Cossio D, Faskowitz J, Santander T, Handwerker DA, et al. Neuroanatomical changes observed over the course of a human pregnancy. Nat Neurosci. 2024 Sep 16;1–8.

62. O'Donoghue K. Fetal microchimerism and maternal health during and after pregnancy. Obstet Med. 2008 Dec;1(2):56–64.

63. Crespi BJ. Why and How Imprinted Genes Drive Fetal Programming. Frontiers in Endocrinology [Internet]. 2020;10. Available from: https://www.frontiersin.org/articles/10.3389/fendo.2019.00940

64. Haig D. Genomic imprinting and kinship: how good is the evidence? Annusl Review of Genetics. 2004;38:553–85.

65. Häyry M, Sukenick A. Imposing a Lifestyle: A New Argument for Antinatalism. Cambridge Quarterly of Healthcare Ethics. 2024 Apr;33(2):238–59.

66. Lopez-Tello J, Yong HEJ, Sandovici I, Dowsett GKC, Christoforou ER, Salazar-Petres E, et al. Fetal manipulation of maternal metabolism is a critical function of the imprinted Igf2 gene. Cell Metabolism. 2023 Jul 11;35(7):1195-1208.e6.

67. News N. Unborn Babies "Remote-Control" Moms for Nutrition via Paternal Gene [Internet]. Neuroscience News. 2023 [cited 2023 Jul 16]. Available from: https://neurosciencenews.com/paternal-genetics-baby-nutrition-23638/

68. David HP. Born Unwanted, 35 Years Later: The Prague Study. Reproductive Health Matters. 2006;14(27):181–90.

69. Foster DG. The Turnaway Study: the cost of denying women access to abortion. New York: Simon and Schuster; 2020.

70. Feldmar A. The embryology of consciousness: What is a normal pregnancy. The psychological aspects of abortion. 1979;15–24.

71. Sonne JC. Interpreting the dread of being aborted in therapy. Journal of Prenatal & Perinatal Psychology & Health. 1997;11(4):185.

72. Sieff DF. The death mother as nature's shadow: Infanticide, abandonment, and the collective unconscious. Psychological Perspectives. 2019;62(1):15–34.

73. Chowdhury A, Islam I, Lee D. The Great Recession, jobs and social crises: policies matter. International Journal of Social Economics. 2013 Jan 1;40(3):220–45.

74. Wu J, Dean KS, Rosen Z, Muennig PA. The cost-effectiveness analysis of nurse-family partnership in the United States. Journal of health care for the poor and underserved. 2017;28(4):1578–97.

75. Steele H, Steele M, Fonagy P. Associations among attachment classifications of mothers, fathers, and their infants. Child Development. 1996;67(2):541–55.

76. Kim S, Fonagy P, Allen J, Martinez S, Iyengar U, Strathearn L. Mothers who are securely attached in pregnancy show more attuned infant mirroring 7 months postpartum. Infant Behavior and Development. 2014;37(4):491–504.

77. Lowell AF, Dell J, Potenza MN, Strathearn L, Mayes LC, Rutherford HJ. Adult attachment is related to maternal neural response to infant cues: an ERP study. Attachment & human development. 2021;1–18.

78. De Rooij SR, Bleker LS, Painter RC, Ravelli AC, Roseboom TJ. Lessons learned from 25 Years of Research into Long term Consequences of Prenatal Exposure to the Dutch famine 1944–45: The Dutch famine Birth Cohort. International Journal of Environmental Health Research. 2022 Jul 3;32(7):1432–46.

79. Barker D. The best start in life. London: Century. 2003;

80. Sandman CA, Davis EP, Glynn LM. Prescient human fetuses thrive. Psychological science. 2012;23(1):93–100.

81. Davis EP, Narayan AJ. Pregnancy as a period of risk, adaptation, and resilience for mothers and infants. Development and Psychopathology. 2020 Dec;32(5):1625–39.

82. Kim S, Deng Q, Fleisher BM, Li S. The Lasting Impact of Parental Early Life Malnutrition on Their Offspring: Evidence from the China Great Leap Forward Famine. World Development. 2014 Feb;54:232–42.

83. Srichaikul K, Hegele RA, Jenkins DJA. Great Chinese Famine and the Effects on Cardiometabolic Health for Future Generations. Hypertension. 2022 Mar;79(3):532–5.

84. Kwon EJ, Kim YJ. What is fetal programming?: a lifetime health is under the control of in utero health. Obstet Gynecol Sci. 2017 Nov;60(6):506–19.

85. Baker BH, Freije S, MacDonald JW, Bammler TK, Benson C, Carroll KN, et al. Placental transcriptomic signatures of prenatal and preconceptional maternal stress. Mol Psychiatry. 2024 Jan 11;1–13.

86. Apanasewicz A, Danel DP, Piosek M, Wychowaniec P, Babiszewska-Aksamit M, Ziomkiewicz A. Maternal childhood trauma is associated with offspring body size during the first year of life. Sci Rep [Internet]. 2022 Nov 15;12(1). Available from: https://www.nature.com/articles/s41598-022-23740-6

87. Zhang Q, Wang Z, Zhang W, Wen Q, Li X, Zhou J, et al. The memory of neuronal mitochondrial stress is inherited transgenerationally via elevated mitochondrial

DNA levels. Nature Cell Biology. 2021;23(8):870–80.

88. Scorza P, Duarte CS, Lee S, Wu H, Posner J, Baccarelli A, et al. Epigenetic Intergenerational Transmission: Mothers' Adverse Childhood Experiences and DNA Methylation. Journal of the American Academy of Child & Adolescent Psychiatry [Internet]. 2023 Jun 15; Available from: https://www.sciencedirect.com/science/article/pii/S0890856723003131

89. Zhu Y, Zhang G, Anme T. Intergenerational associations of adverse and positive maternal childhood experiences with young children's psychosocial well-being. Eur J Psychotraumatol. 14(1):2185414.

90. Selye H. The stress of life. New York: McGraw-Hill; 1956.

91. Eberle C, Fasig T, Brüseke F, Stichling S. Impact of maternal prenatal stress by glucocorticoids on metabolic and cardiovascular outcomes in their offspring: a systematic scoping review. PloS one. 2021;16(1).

92. DiPietro JA, Novak MFSX, Costigan KA, Atella LD, Reusing SP. Maternal Psychological Distress During Pregnancy in Relation to Child Development at Age Two. Child Development. 2006;77(3):573–87.

93. Gerhardt S. Why love matters: How affection shapes a baby's brain. London: Routledge; 2004.

94. Glover V, O'Donnell KJ, O'Connor TG, Fisher J. Prenatal maternal stress, fetal programming, and mechanisms underlying later psychopathology—a global perspective. Development and psychopathology. 2018;30(3):843–54.

95. Zanetti D, Tikkanen E, Gustafsson S, Priest JR, Burgess S, Ingelsson E. Birthweight, Type 2 Diabetes Mellitus, and Cardiovascular Disease. Circulation: Genomic and Precision Medicine [Internet]. 2018 Jun;11(6). Available from: https://www.ahajournals.org/doi/full/10.1161/CIRCGEN.117.002054

96. Barker DJP. The Developmental Origins of Chronic Disease. In: Landale NS, McHale SM, Booth A, editors. Families and Child Health. Springer New York; 2013. p. 3–11. (National Symposium on Family Issues).

97. Lou HC, Hansen D, Nordentoft M, Pryds O, Jensen F, Nim J, et al. Prenatal stressors of human life affect fetal brain development. Developmental Medicine & Child Neurology. 1994;36(9):826–32.

98. Kofman O. The role of prenatal stress in the etiology of developmental behavioural disorders. Neuroscience & Biobehavioral Reviews. 2002;26(4):457–70.

99. Thornburg KL, Boone-Heinonen J, Valent AM. Social Determinants of Placental Health and Future Disease Risks for Babies. Obstetrics and Gynecology Clinics of North America. 2020 Mar 1;47(1):1–15.

100. Atzl VM, Narayan AJ, Rivera LM, Lieberman AF. Adverse childhood experiences and prenatal mental health: Type of ACEs and age of maltreatment onset. Journal of family psychology. 2019;33(3):304–14.

101. Manzari N, Matvienko-Sikar K, Baldoni F, O'Keeffe GW, Khashan AS. Prenatal maternal stress and risk of neurodevelopmental disorders in the offspring: a systematic review and meta-analysis. Soc Psychiatry Psychiatr Epidemiol. 2019 Nov 1;54(11):1299–309.

102. Nazzari S, Fearon P, Rice F, Ciceri F, Molteni M, Frigerio A. Neuroendocrine and immune markers of maternal stress during pregnancy and infant cognitive

development. Developmental Psychobiology. 2020;62(8):1100–10.

103. Nazzari S, Fearon P, Rice F, Dottori N, Ciceri F, Molteni M, et al. Beyond the HPA-axis: Exploring maternal prenatal influences on birth outcomes and stress reactivity. Psychoneuroendocrinology. 2019 Mar 1;101:253–62.

104. Sacchi C, De Carli P, Gregorini C, Monk C, Simonelli A. In the pandemic from the womb. Prenatal exposure, maternal psychological stress and mental health in association with infant negative affect at 6 months of life. Dev Psychopathol. 2023 Feb 16;1–11.

105. Grande LA, Swales DA, Sandman CA, Glynn LM, Davis EP. Maternal caregiving ameliorates the consequences of prenatal maternal psychological distress on child development. Development and Psychopathology. 2022 Oct;34(4):1376–85.

106. Okano L, Ji Y, Riley AW, Wang X. Maternal psychosocial stress and children's ADHD diagnosis: a prospective birth cohort study. Journal of Psychosomatic Obstetrics & Gynecology. 2019;40(3):217–25.

107. Olds DL. Improving the Life Chances of Vulnerable Children and Families with Prenatal and Infancy Support of Parents: The Nurse-Family Partnership*. Psychosocial Intervention. 2012;21(2):129–43.

108. Scorza P, Monk C. Anticipating the stork: Stress and trauma during pregnancy and the importance of prenatal parenting. Zero to Three. 2020;

109. Foley S, Hughes C, Fink E. Expectant mothers' not fathers' mind-mindedness predicts infant, mother, and father conversational turns at 7 months. Infancy. 2022;27(6):1091–103.

110. Zhang W, Rajendran K, Ham J, Finik J, Buthmann J, Davey K, et al. Prenatal exposure to disaster-related traumatic stress and developmental trajectories of temperament in early childhood: Superstorm Sandy pregnancy study. Journal of affective disorders. 2018;234:335–45.

111. Walsh K, McCormack CA, Webster R, Pinto A, Lee S, Feng T, et al. Maternal prenatal stress phenotypes associate with fetal neurodevelopment and birth outcomes. Proceedings of the National Academy of Sciences. 2019 Nov 26;116(48):23996–4005.

112. Roe KV, Drivas A. Planned conception and infant functioning at age three months: A cross-cultural study. American Journal of Orthopsychiatry. 1993;63(1):120–5.

113. Takács L, Štipl J, Gartstein M, Putnam SP, Monk C. Social support buffers the effects of maternal prenatal stress on infants' unpredictability. Early Human Development. 2021 Jun 1;157:105352.

114. Yuda IP, Yuwindry I, Anggrita S. Side Effects of Antidepressant Drug Use During Pregnancy: Literature Review. International Conference on Health and Science. 2021 Nov 1;1(1):824–40.

115. Heinonen E, Forsberg L, Nörby U, Wide K, Källén K. Neonatal morbidity after fetal exposure to antipsychotics: a national register-based study. BMJ Open [Internet]. 2022;12(6). Available from:
https://bmjopen.bmj.com/content/12/6/e061328

116. Barry JM, Birnbaum AK, Jasin LR, Sherwin CM. Maternal Exposure and Neonatal Effects of Drugs of Abuse. The Journal of Clinical Pharmacology. 2021;61(S2):142–55.

117. Emanuel R. Psychotherapy with children traumatized in infancy. Journal of Child Psychotherapy. 1996;22(2):214–39.

118. Wozniak JR, Riley EP, Charness ME. Clinical presentation, diagnosis, and management of fetal alcohol spectrum disorder. The Lancet Neurology. 2019;18(8):760–70.

119. Mattson SN, Bernes GA, Doyle LR. Fetal alcohol spectrum disorders: a review of the neurobehavioral deficits associated with prenatal alcohol exposure. Alcoholism: Clinical and Experimental Research. 2019;43(6):1046–62.

120. Cambiasso MY, Gotfryd L, Stinson MG, Birolo S, Salamone G, Romanato M, et al. Paternal alcohol consumption has intergenerational consequences in male offspring. Journal of Assisted Reproduction and Genetics. 2022;39(2):441–59.

121. Margolis AE, Liu R, Conceição VA, Ramphal B, Pagliaccio D, DeSerisy ML, et al. Convergent neural correlates of prenatal exposure to air pollution and behavioral phenotypes of risk for internalizing and externalizing problems: Potential biological and cognitive pathways. Neuroscience & Biobehavioral Reviews [Internet]. 2022 Jun 1;137. Available from: https://www.sciencedirect.com/science/article/pii/S0149763422001348

122. Carrington D, editor DCE. Microplastics found in every human testicle in study. The Guardian [Internet]. 2024 May 20 [cited 2024 Jun 12]; Available from: https://www.theguardian.com/environment/article/2024/may/20/microplastics-human-testicles-study-sperm-counts

123. Wadman E, Fernandes E, Muss C, Powell-Hamilton N, Wojcik MH, Madden JA, et al. A novel syndrome associated with prenatal fentanyl exposure. Genetics in Medicine Open. 2023 Jan 1;1(1):100834.

124. Pregnancy, breastfeeding and fertility while using fentanyl [Internet]. nhs.uk. 2023 [cited 2024 Aug 17]. Available from: https://www.nhs.uk/medicines/fentanyl/pregnancy-breastfeeding-and-fertility-while-using-fentanyl/

125. Margolis AE, Lee SH, Liu R, Goolsby L, Champagne F, Herbstman J, et al. Associations between prenatal exposure to second hand smoke and infant self-regulation in a New York city longitudinal prospective birth cohort. Environ Res. 2023 Jun 15;227:115652.

126. Glover V. Prenatal mental health and the effects of stress on the foetus and the child. Should psychiatrists look beyond mental disorders? World Psychiatry. 2020;19(3):331–2.

127. Leve LD, Neiderhiser JM, Harold GT, Natsuaki MN, Bohannan BJM, Cresko WA. Naturalistic Experimental Designs as Tools for Understanding the Role of Genes and the Environment in Prevention Research. Prev Sci. 2018 Jan 1;19(1):68–78.

128. Lacey RE, Howe LD, Kelly-Irving M, Bartley M, Kelly Y. The Clustering of Adverse Childhood Experiences in the Avon Longitudinal Study of Parents and Children: J Interpers Violence. 2022 Mar 1;37(5–6):2218–41.

129. Hilmert CJ, Dominguez TP, Schetter CD, Srinivas SK, Glynn LM, Hobel CJ, et al. Lifetime racism and blood pressure changes during pregnancy: Implications for fetal growth. Health Psychology. 2014;33(1):43–51.

130. Weissman DG, Hatzenbuehler ML, Cikara M, Barch DM, McLaughlin KA. State-level macro-economic factors moderate the association of low income with brain

structure and mental health in U.S. children. Nat Commun. 2023 May 2;14(1):2085.

131. Kram JJF, Montgomery MO, Moreno ACP, Romdenne TA, Forgie MM. Family-centered cesarean delivery: American Journal of Obstetrics & Gynecology MFM [Internet]. 2021 Nov 1;3(6).

132. Pavličev M, Romero R, Mitteroecker P. Evolution of the human pelvis and obstructed labor: new explanations of an old obstetrical dilemma. American Journal of Obstetrics and Gynecology. 2020 Jan 1;222(1):3–16.

133. Dunsworth HM. There Is No "Obstetrical Dilemma": Towards a Braver Medicine with Fewer Childbirth Interventions. Perspect Biol Med. 2018;61(2):249–63.

134. Shen X, Bagherigaleh S. Acupuncture and Pregnancy: Classical Meets Modern. Medical Acupuncture. 2019 Oct;31(5):248–50.

135. Odent M. Is the participation of the father at birth dangerous? Midwifery Today Int Midwife. 1999;(51):23–4.

136. Sargent C. Obstetrical choice among urban women in Benin. Social Science & Medicine. 1985;20(3):287–92.

137. Klaus MH, Kennell JH, Klaus PH. Mothering the mother: how a doula can help you have a shorter, easier, and healthier birth. Reading MA: Perseus; 1993.

138. Hildingsson I, Karlström A, Larsson B. Childbirth experience in women participating in a continuity of midwifery care project. Women and Birth. 2021 May 1;34(3):e255–61.

139. MacKinnon AL, Houazene S, Robins S, Feeley N, Zelkowitz P. Maternal Attachment Style, Interpersonal Trauma History, and Childbirth-Related Post-traumatic Stress. Frontiers in Psychology, 2018;9.

140. Balaskas J. Active birth-revised Edition: the new approach to giving birth naturally. Harvard Common Press; 1992.

141. Wilson DR. Hypnobirthing. International Journal of Childbirth Education. 2017;32(4).

142. Bardacke N. Mindful birthing: training the mind, body, and heart for childbirth and beyond. New York: Harper Collins; 2012.

143. Webb R, Bond R, Romero-Gonzalez B, Mycroft R, Ayers S. Interventions to treat fear of childbirth in pregnancy: a systematic review and meta-analysis. Psychological Medicine. 2021 Sep;51(12):1964–77.

144. Sobczak A, Taylor L, Solomon S, Ho J, Kemper S, Phillips B, et al. The Effect of Doulas on Maternal and Birth Outcomes: A Scoping Review. Cureus. 15(5):e39451.

145. Campos-Berga L, Moreno-Giménez A, Vento M, Diago V, Hervás D, Sáenz P, et al. Cumulative life stressors and stress response to threatened preterm labour as birth date predictors. Arch Gynecol Obstet. 2022 Jun 1;305(6):1421–9.

146. Hodnett ED, Gates S, Hofmeyr GJ, Sakala C. Continuous support for women during childbirth (Review). The Cochrane database of systematic reviews. 2007;3.

147. Cankaya S, Can R. The effect of continuous supportive care on birth pain, birth fear, midwifery care perception, oxytocin use, and delivery time during the intrapartum period. Nigerian Journal of Clinical Practice [Internet]. 2021 Jan 11;24(11)

148. Braveman P, Dominguez TP, Burke W, Dolan SM, Stevenson DK, Jackson FM, et al. Explaining the Black-White Disparity in Preterm Birth. Frontiers in

Reproductive Health [Internet]. 2021

149. Young M, Thomas M. Wordsmith: The Gift of a Soul. Faversham: Medlar Tree Publishing; 2013. 96 p.

150. Simpson M, Schmied V, Dickson C, Dahlen HG. Postnatal post-traumatic stress: An integrative review. Women and Birth. 2018 Oct 1;31(5):367–79.

151. Keedle H, Willo MP. P18 - Using poetic inquiry to give voice to women who had a traumatic birth through bearing witness. Women and Birth. 2022 Sep 1;35:47–8.

152. Birth Trauma, Obstetric Violence and Birth Rape – ISSTD News [Internet]. [cited 2023 Aug 25]. Available from: https://news.isst-d.org/birth-trauma-obstetric-violence-and-birth-rape/

153. Svanberg E. Why Birth Trauma Matters. London: Pinter & Martin Limited; 2019. 160 p.

154. Wickham S. Inducing Labour: making informed decisions. 2nd edition. Birthmoon Creations; 2018. 168 p.

155. Murray L, Cooper P. Postpartum Depression and Child Development. New York: Guilford; 1999.

156. Porthan E, Lindberg M, Härkönen J, Scheinin NM, Karlsson L, Karlsson H, et al. Childhood trauma and fear of childbirth: findings from a birth cohort study. Archives of women's mental health. 2023;1–7.

157. Limb M. Disparity in maternal deaths because of ethnicity is "unacceptable." BMJ. 2021 Jan 18;372:n152.

158. Racial Disparities Persist in Maternal Morbidity, Mortality and Infant Health [Internet]. AJMC. 2020. Available from: https://www.ajmc.com/view/racial-disparities-persist-in-maternal-morbidity-mortality-and-infant-health

159. Markin RD, Coleman MN. Intersections of gendered racial trauma and childbirth trauma: Clinical interventions for Black women. Psychotherapy. 2023;60(1):27.

INDEX

A

abortion, 14, 39, 73-75, 153, 154

abuse, 75, 82, 91, 95, 96, 126, 127, 131, 132, 135, 150, 152, 156

Active Birth Movement, 108

adrenaline, 5, 107

Adult Attachment Interview (AAI), 78

adverse childhood experiences (ACEs), 9, 85, 113, 142, 150, 155, 157

Akilapa, Nikita, viii, 45, 52, 56, 102, 124, 133

ambivalence, 8, 48, 55, 67, 72, 73, 75, 76

amniotic fluid, 8, 22, 25, 26

ancestral tradition, 42, 104

ancient rituals, 141

Andean tribes, 65

anti-depressants, 92

anti-psychotics, 93, 156

antinatalism, 71, 153

APGAR score, 122

attachment, x, 40-44, 46, 47, 78-80, 92, 107, 144, 148, 149, 152, 154, 158

autoimmune issues, 69

B

Barbieri, Annalisa, iii, viii

Barker, David, 36, 81, 88

Bateson, Dr Karen, iii

beta-endorphins, 107

Bick, Esther, 29

Big Pharma, 94

binge eating, 82

biological sex, xv, 19

birth complications, 52, 88, 91, 92, 107, 137

birth trauma, 39, 122, 126, 128, 130, 159

birthgiver, xv, 9, 15, 42-44, 48, 50, 109, 141

birthing stories, 105

black women, 113, 133, 159

blastocyst, 15

Bowlby, John, 40

Bowlby's psychoanalytic contemporaries, 42

Helen Deutsch, 42

Therese Benedek, 42

brain areas, 35, 93, 94

brain inflammation, 94

160

hippocampus, 35, 94

brain-derived neurotrophic factor (BDNF), 94

brain-wave signals, 50

alpha, 50

delta, 50

breastfeeding, 74, 91, 107, 112, 130, 135, 157

breathing and movements, 29

breech position, 52

British Birth Trauma Association, 128

C

c-section, 110, 111, 120, 129

caesarean section, 56, 99-101, 107, 111, 128

cardiovascular disease, 82, 155

cerebellum, 34, 35

cerebral cortex, 35

cerebrum, 34, 35

Chamberlain, David, 9, 142

Chown, Annabel, viii, 4, 49, 78, 110

co-embodiment, 23, 69, 142

co-operative breeding species, 41

co-regulation, 8, 142

cocaine, 24, 37

conception, 6, 9, 12-14, 33, 61, 69, 83, 140, 150, 154, 156

Condon, John, 43

coronary heart disease, 88

corticosteroids, 27

cortisol level, 87, 89, 91

Cuna of Panama, 61

D

Dagara people of Burkina Faso, 61

Dalton, Katharina, 34

Dendrites, 35

diabetes, 24, 70, 88, 155

dizygotic, 29

DNA changes (see also methylation), 85

Dogon people of Mali, 64

doula, 10, 45, 107, 111, 112, 118, 122-125, 130, 134, 139, 143, 158

Dunsworth, Holly, 100

dysmorphic facial features, 93

dysregulated nervous system, 91

E

Efe, 41, 152

embryo (see also epiblast), 4, 14, 15, 57, 68, 69, 83

enzyme, 88

epiblast, 15

Epidural, 111, 121, 127

epigenetic history, 9, 142

episiotomy, 134

Eurocentric, 62

F

fallopian tube, 15

Family Nurse Partnership, 75, 90

family-centred caesarean birth, 99

Feldmar, Andrew, 73

fentanyl, 94, 157

first trimester, 17, 18, 24, 32, 34, 61, 105

fMRIs, 90

foetal alcohol spectrum disorder (FASD), 93

foetal alcohol syndrome (FAS), 94

foetal position, 27

foetal programming, 36, 81, 83

foetus, I, iii-v, xii, 2, 3, 6-11, 13-15, 17-29, 32, 35, 36, 40, 42-44, 46-51, 53-57, 61-63, 65, 68-72, 75-77, 80-84, 86-93, 95, 107, 108, 140-143, 153m 157

Fonagy, Peter, x, 78

Four D scans, 24, 28, 32, 45

G

genes, 3, 9, 68, 70, 71, 72, 84, 85, 88, 95, 153, 157

genome, 29, 71, 141

gentle C-section, 99

German measles (see also rubella), 34

gestational diabetes, 70

gluconeogenesis, 84

Gottlieb, Alma, 53

Granville, Scarlett, 129

grey matter, 35

H

habituation, 23

Haig, David, 71

Hausa in Nigeria, 54

hCG, 15

heroin-addicted newborns, 93

Himba of Namibia, 103

hippocampus, 35, 94,

home birth, 101, 115, 124

homeostasis, 8, 150

hormones, 5, 13, 30, 68, 70, 84, 129

human chorionic gonadotropin, hCG, 15

hypnobirthing, 108, 110, 124, 158

I

Igbo tribesmen of Nigeria, 61

in vitro fertilisation (IVF), 95

Indigenous Australian women, 103

Indigenous knowledge, v, 7, 59, 141

induction, 100, 110, 116, 127-130, 138

infant observation, 29, 151

inflammatory issues, 113

intergenerational trauma, 142

intrauterine environment, 8, 22, 27,